CAREER CHOICES FOR VETERINARIANS

Beyond Private Practice

OTHER BOOKS BY CARIN A. SMITH, DVM

THE RELIEF VETERINARIAN'S MANUAL
(And Survival Guide)
Smith Veterinary Services 1990, rev. 1997

THE HOUSECALL VETERINARIAN'S MANUAL
Smith Veterinary Services 1996, rev.1997

THE EMPLOYER'S GUIDE TO HIRING
RELIEF AND PART-TIME DVMs
Smith Veterinary Services 1993, rev. 1997

GET RID OF FLEAS AND TICKS FOR GOOD!
Smith Veterinary Services 1995

101 TRAINING TIPS FOR YOUR CAT
Dell Publishing 1994

EASY HEALTH CARE FOR YOUR HORSE
Simon & Schuster / Prentice-Hall 1991

CAREER CHOICES FOR VETERINARIANS

Beyond Private Practice

Carin A. Smith, DVM

SMITH VETERINARY SERVICES

Leavenworth, Washington

CAREER CHOICES FOR VETERINARIANS
Beyond Private Practice

CARIN A. SMITH, DVM

Published by
Smith Veterinary Services
PO Box 254, Leavenworth WA 98826 USA

Cover design and illustration by Lightbourne Images, © 1997

First edition, 1998

Smith, Carin
Career Choices for Veterinarians: Beyond Private Practice
Carin A. Smith. 1st ed.
    Includes bibliographical references and index.
    ISBN 1-885780-08-7

Publisher's Cataloging in Publication Data

Smith, Carin A.
Career Choices for Veterinarians: Beyond Private Practice / Carin A. Smith
p.   cm.
Includes bibliographical references and index.
ISBN 1-885780-08-7
1. Veterinary medicine—Vocational guidance. 2. Veterinary medicine.
3. Vocational guidance. I. Title.
SF756.28.S65x
636.089'023   Library of Congress Catalog Card Number
                                                    97-91960

ACKNOWLEDGMENTS

Gathering information for this book took two years and involved interviews with veterinarians all over the United States—and the world.

A heartfelt *thank you* to all the veterinarians, company representatives, and government officials who answered my inquiries about veterinary jobs.

Additional thanks goes to those who were gracious enough to review the manuscript draft and offer constructive criticism. You have my deepest gratitude.

FOREWORD

It was a distinct privilege to be asked to review this book, given that the author is a person who I know to be thorough, meticulous, and pleasantly exuberant as well as deadly serious in any writing project she undertakes. Perhaps Dr. Smith's greatest attribute as a gifted writer is that she knows how to do exhaustive research on the subject she intends to address. Readers of any of her many dissertations can rest assured that what gets into print is up to date and authoritative. I do not have the broad perspective to pass unequivocal judgment on that score in this particular book, but from my experience in working with her in the past, I have faith that this book will not lead any reader down a primrose path.

Dr. Smith is a consummate artist in describing the advantages and disadvantages of any course of action that might be taken in the professional arena, without offending anyone whose strong viewpoint might contrast with that of anyone else, as she did so well when she wrote commissioned "Research Roundup" articles for the Journal of the AVMA for several years. In this book, she does the same, as she offers "Pros and Cons" of various job opportunities—only one of the many features of the book that provides helpful insights beyond what might be inferred between the lines.

Dr. Smith's intended reading audience (veterinarians and those considering a veterinary career) will get a more-than-worthwhile bang for the buck, for no stone is left unturned. Indeed, some of the job descriptions seemed excessively detailed, at least for veterinarians who have been around awhile and keep current with the world about them. I am confident, though, that readers who aspire to a veterinary career or who may be recent graduates looking for a more satisfying career pathway will absorb the wealth of information like a sponge.

Last, but certainly not least, Dr. Smith's superlative writing skill should serve to underscore the all-important point she emphasizes throughout the book—that those who aspire to positions of leadership and considerable responsibility in the veterinary profession may not reach the pinnacle of success unless they first master effective oral and written communication skills. Dr. Smith, I am proud to say, has done that exceedingly well, as exemplified in this, her latest, literary work. Let us hope that her energy never flags, and that many more good books spring from her keyboard through her love affair with words and the abundance of useful information that surely will be derivable therefrom.

—*Dr. Albert J. Koltveit, retired editor-in-chief (1984-1995), American Veterinary Medical Association*

CONTENTS

INTRODUCTION

WHO SHOULD READ THIS BOOK?

- Veterinarians

- Those considering a veterinary career

Whether you're a seasoned veterinarian, a new graduate, or an aspiring veterinarian, you will find a wide array of career pathways available to you. After a review of "traditional" practice, you'll get to the interesting part—career choices beyond private practice. *The careers discussed here focus on those that don't require any degree beyond that of* DVM.

Students: Some of you may have already decided on your area of interest in veterinary medicine, while others wonder about new choices you've not yet considered. Either way, you'll gain from taking a fresh look at your chosen career. Perhaps you'll realize that you would be smart to get a Bachelors degree in business to best prepare for veterinary school, or you may change your thoughts about the type of externships you want to take as a veterinary student. You may realize that you'd be smart to take a summer job in a research lab or in a public health department in order to add "research experience" or "epidemiology" to your resume. Broadening your horizons will only enrich your opportunities.

Veterinarians: You're the ones who will truly gain from this information. Some of you may be new veterinary school graduates who are exploring all your options before you select a job. Perhaps you are an experienced veterinarian who, after four years of veterinary school and several years of practice, are disconcerted to realize that you are not fully satisfied. Maybe you're an employee in a practice, with no hope or desire to buy in as an owner. Or perhaps you already own a practice, but have not found the satisfaction you desire, and your personal life is suffering. Even veterinarians who have enjoyed their private practice careers may be interested in a change. After all, those who graduate from veterinary school at age 25 can potentially look forward to 40-50 years of work. Why spend it all doing the same thing?

For many veterinarians, the problem is financial need. The average starting salary for 1996 grads was around $33,500—with an average debt of $49,000. The income per DVM is expected to decline over the next decade. After spending all your savings and going into debt to complete veterinary school, you may have difficulty finding a job in private practice that pays adequately, especially if you are limited geographically by family or other constraints. What's more, the cost of buying into or starting your own veterinary hospital is out of reach of many veterinarians. Yet life as an employee in private practice is not always an ideal long-term career. The choice needn't be "either/or" when it comes to making a good living and having a job you enjoy.

Most veterinary students get a short "review" of "alternative careers" in school. If your review was like mine, you left the class knowing that you could work in industry, government, or private practice, or that you could further your schooling and become a specialist. But no one told us, in an organized and detailed manner, about all the opportunities that exist within those categories. So we left with our own stereotypic views of "industry" and "government" jobs. After reading this book, you will find out what choices really exist.

With that in mind, take this advice:

Dismiss all job stereotypes from your mind, and read the entire book before you start to narrow your choices.

Seek out veterinarians who have non-traditional jobs and ask them about their work. Talk to people with jobs you think you won't like—you may be pleasantly surprised.

BEFORE YOU DIVE IN

Using resource lists

As you read, you will see references to books, articles, or online sources of further information. You will find a "resource list" in each section and chapter of the book, as well as a general resource list in the Appendix, with resources that apply to many job situations. These resources include groups affiliated with each job category; places to find job announcements; Web sites that provide information, job applications, and links to related material; phone numbers and E-mail addresses; and books and articles. Don't let yourself get stalled by being unable to access those information sources.

Format of E-mail addresses and Web sites

An E-mail address is one that you can write to. Its form will be something like this: smithvet@nwinternet.com

A Web site (or "home page") is a collection of information available online that you can view using your modem and Internet-access software. Web sites offer a wide variety of information, including job announcements and free literature for business owners. A Web address (or URL, Uniform Resource Locator) will look something like this: http://www.now2000.com/smithvet

In this book, we've omitted the words "phone" before phone numbers, "address" before street addresses, "E-mail" before electronic mail addresses, and "Web site" before Web site addresses. You know what each one is from its form.

Thus a typical resource listing might be:

Smith Veterinary Services, PO Box 254, Leavenworth WA 98826; 509-763-2052; Fax 509-763-2112; smithvet@nwinternet.com http://www.now2000.com/smithvet

Every attempt has been made to include current information. However, many groups use their President's address as their only contact point. To find the current address, look in the *AVMA Membership Directory and Resource Manual,* (see Appendix) or search for the group by its name on the Web.

Accessing Web sites and online services

The world is computerized. Are you? *I can't stress enough how much easier your career search is going to be if you have access to online services.* Instead of making several phone calls and being bounced around; instead of writing hundreds of letters and waiting for replies, only to have to send out more letters to other departments; instead of getting job announcements weeks after they've been published; instead of spending all that money on postage, envelopes, and paper—instead of all that, you can get instant information at low cost simply by using a computer and modem to access the Internet and the World Wide Web.

If you aren't yet online, consider the purchase of a computer and modem, and the investment of learning time, as a huge part of your career search. Not only will your search be easier, you will now be able to say you have basic computer skills! Get a friend to help you hook up. Read *PC World* magazine to find out what computer systems are best.

In addition to the Web sites listed in each book chapter, see the Appendix for a list of Web sites that include job announcements.

Internet addresses may change. If you try to go to a Web site and find that it has disappeared, don't give up. Write to the group's street address, or use an online search engine to find the group's new Web address.

A good review of online services, including basic definitions of terms, can be found in:

Veterinary Medical Resources on the Internet. John Dascanio et al. The Compendium on Continuing Education for the Practicing Veterinarian. 19(2) 2/97 pp 205-212.

Obtaining books and articles mentioned in this book

It is unlikely that you will find many of the books or articles listed here just by looking in your local library or bookstore. That isn't a big problem, though.

Borrowing books

I suggest ordering any book of interest from your nearby public library. Then, if you find it particularly helpful, you may decide to buy it later. Don't worry if your library doesn't have a particular book on its shelves or in its catalog. Just ask the librarian to order a copy through the interlibrary loan service. Some libraries may charge a small fee for this service.

Purchasing books

First you need to find out whether the book is still in print. If not, you'll have to order it from the library. (Being out of print has nothing to do with a book's quality—the nature of the publishing business is such that books go out of print quickly.) To find out whether a book is in print, just call any local bookstore. They can look in their computer to find the title, then can order it for you. You can also order books online through a variety of bookstores, such as Amazon.
http://www.amazon.com

Ordering copies of articles

You can get copies of articles two ways: by ordering reprints from the magazine, or by ordering reprints from your library. Your library needn't have a particular magazine or journal on its shelves in order to get you a copy of an article. Just ask the librarian to order the copy through the interlibrary loan service.

Some library systems perform this service at no charge; if yours does, that's the best way to go. Other libraries charge a fee; if that's the case, check with the magazine and compare their reprint fee with the fee the library charges. You can also order copies of articles through online services; I've found this to be expensive and slow, but that may change.

Sample job announcements and pay ranges

Various sections of this book include samples of job announcements to give you an idea of the type of work and qualifications required for various jobs. Obviously, they are not current announcements, but it is possible that similar openings are available. Contact the appropriate agency for current job announcements. Likewise, pay ranges are not current but serve as a guideline to let you know the approximate pay you could expect. Salaries listed, when available, are those for 1996-1997.

Accuracy note

A great effort was made to gather accurate information for this book during an exhaustive, 2-year search. However, agencies and organizations continually change their internal structures or job descriptions. What's more, there were not official job descriptions for some positions, and some of my inquiries went unanswered. Much of the information presented here was obtained from interviews with individuals who described their specific positions. It is possible that occasional inaccuracies exist in the text, and it's also likely that additional job opportunities exist that are not mentioned here. Contact the groups or hiring agencies listed in each resource list for complete and timely information.

Abbreviations and terms

All veterinarians will be familiar with the terms used in this book. Students may want to keep a pocket dictionary handy for looking up the occasional mysterious word.

"Career choices"

"I thought veterinary medicine *was* a career!"

The traditional veterinary career is one in private practice, with other types of jobs usually being considered "alternatives" to that. However, the American Veterinary Medical Association (AVMA) has indicated that it wants to discourage the use of "alternate career pathways" or similar phrases and instead encourage the use of the phrase, "practice fields in veterinary medicine."

A career, in my mind, is a job pathway that a person takes over a long period. When I speak of a "career choice" in this book, I mean a job or series of jobs that become a long-term occupation, still within the field of veterinary medicine. I've used the words "career" and "job" interchangeably with "career field," "career pathway," or "practice field."

Many jobs discussed here are temporary or short-term positions such as fellowships, volunteer opportunities, or one-year positions. These jobs, in addition to the option of returning to school, can all be a part of your career.

"DVM"

As a convenience, I've used the abbreviation "DVM" throughout this book in place of the word "veterinarian." This is in no way meant to slight Pennsylvania graduates, who receive a VMD degree, or foreign graduates, who receive an ECFVG certificate to practice in the US.

Frequently-used abbreviations

AAAS American Association for the Advancement of Science
AAHA American Animal Hospital Association
AJVR American Journal of Veterinary Research
APHIS Animal and Plant Health Inspection Service
ARS Agricultural Research Service
AVMA American Veterinary Medical Association
CDC Centers For Disease Control and Prevention
CE continuing education
CEAH Centers for Epidemiology and Animal Health
CV curriculum vitae
CVM Center for Veterinary Medicine
DVM Doctor of Veterinary Medicine
ECFVG Educational Commission for Foreign Veterinary Graduates
EPA Environmental Protection Agency
FAO Food and Agriculture Organization
FDA Food and Drug Administration
FSIS Food Safety and Inspection Service
FWS Fish and Wildlife Service

HSS US Dept of Health and Human Services
JAVMA Journal of the American Veterinary Medical Association
MPH Masters in Public Health
NIH National Institutes of Health
NSF National Science Foundation
OPM Office of Personnel Management (Federal)
ORACBA Office of Risk Assessment and Cost-Benefit Analysis
OSHA Occupational Safety & Health Administration
PAHO Pan American Health Organization
PHS Public Health Service
PVPCP Public Veterinary Practice Career Program (APHIS)
UN United Nations
USAID United States Dept of State, Agency for International Development
USDA United States Dept of Agriculture
WHO World Health Organization

CHAPTER 1

ORGANIZE YOUR JOB SEARCH

SECRETS OF SUCCESS: HOW TO APPLY FOR ANY JOB

There are two methods of applying for any job: The "official written description of how to apply" and the "unofficial tips about how to get the job."

New graduates and practicing DVMs have a good idea of how to find jobs in private practice. These openings are advertised in state veterinary newsletters and nationally distributed veterinary publications. However, experienced DVMs also know that many private practice jobs are filled by word of mouth or networking. This is also the best way to find jobs outside of private practice. You will get the "official" word on how to apply for a given job in each section of this book. In addition to filling out the proper forms and sending in your resume, there is another approach that works as well or better.

Before you go out and "apply" for a job, take a different approach. Go on an "information gathering" expedition. The purpose of this is twofold: First, to actually gather information; second, to network—that is, to meet lots of people, and let them meet you. These contacts, over time, create a great resource for you.

How do you find these people? Start with the *AVMA Directory*; look up the name and phone number of the nearest extension agent, food inspector, USDA/APHIS DVM, or State Public Health DVM. Call people who are doing the work you're interested in, and ask them if you can make an appointment to come in and talk about their job or their company (or invite them to lunch—you treat). Then do just that. Don't ask for a job, but simply find out as much as you can. Be honest in telling them that you are thinking of changing career pathways, and are gathering information.

Another part of your information gathering and networking is participation in special interest groups. Throughout this book you will see listings of these groups, which vary from the Association of Federal Veterinarians to the Society of Technical Communicators. Find out when these groups meet and attend their conferences. Be ready to introduce yourself and start a conversation. Asking people about themselves is a good start. You will then be able to meet a large number of people working in that field, and will get an in-depth look at the variety of opportunities that may be available.

Make a plan to tackle the exhibit area at a large veterinary meeting. Make your approach while lectures are in session, the exhibit hall is quiet, and exhibitors have the time and interest to talk to you. Prepare ahead of time by taking notes on the exhibits you're interested in—whether that be companies devoted to computer software, pet food, pharmaceuticals, or equipment.

No matter which approach or combination of approaches you take, be sure that you give your business card to everyone you meet. The card need only state your name, phone number and address (include an E-mail address if you have one). You needn't worry about having an official "job title" on the card.

Once you have met a lot of people in different jobs, two things will happen: you'll have a much better idea of what's involved in specific jobs, and people will have met you and will remember you at a later date. (Since you will be meeting a large number of people, make a habit of jotting short notes on their business cards to remind you where you met and what you talked about.)

Now you have the contacts and the information you need to send in your job application. You know a lot about the job you want; you know who to address your letter and application to; and you know what the company needs. When your application crosses the right desk, that person will remember you. If there is a job opening, you might be the first person who comes to mind.

Resources

How to Work a Room. Susan RoAne, Warner Books 1989. Essential reading if you're unsure about this "networking" thing.

Your resume or curriculum vitae

These words can confuse some of you. Most people in the job world use a resume to describe their job history and special talents. Veterinarians in academia are accustomed to using a cv to describe their educational background.

The words "curriculum vitae" mean "class life" or "life study course," and thus the cv is a list of academic accomplishments. It is a document of the course of your studies and everything relevant to them—including all the classes taken, papers or books published, and grants sought and awarded.

A resume is an abstract of the cv plus any job history, skills, and experience that are relevant to the employer. It may include special abilities, honors and awards, and groups or associations to which you belong. The resume is short—one or two pages at most. Use of a resume offers the advantage of adjusting it to suit each situation, while the cv remains as is, adding only further studies or grants.

Many people use a combined resume and cv, where the resume summarizes the attached cv and includes the information that is relevant to the employer's needs, whereas the cv shows only the academic information. The combined cv is better suited to the working professional.

Many books have been written about how to write a successful resume (your local library or bookstore will have at least one choice). Studying those will help you ensure that your resume is the best it can be.

The interview

Imagine you're in an actual interview for a real job opening. To help you relax during the interview, think of it in reverse of the usual way: *You* interview *the employer* to find out whether you want to work for them. If you assume that you are qualified for the job (and you know this because you have done adequate research about the job opening, the company or governmental agency, and their needs), then your approach can only be "of course they will want to hire me," and your goals will be to 1) show them why they need you, i.e., what you can do for them; and 2) find out if you *want* to work for them. (Here's where the pre-job-hunting "information gathering" expedition helps, too. One big worry is "how to dress appropriately." If you've been in that company's office before, you had a chance to see how they dress, and you can match your style to theirs—but err on the dressed-up side.)

One problem that may arise is that you find a job for which you're ideally qualified, but which is not advertised as a job specifically for a veterinarian. You may face the hurdle of changing your interviewer's stereotype of what a veterinarian is, before you will be seriously considered for the job. Unfortunately for veterinary medicine, some veterinarians have found that it is not in their favor to point out that they are veterinarians. Instead, that's just a "by the way" comment, with other qualifications being more important. This may be a necessary strategy for you to use to get a particular job; but if it works, then use your new position to re-educate your colleagues about the wide range of talents found in veterinarians.

The AVMA Career Development Center

Veterinarians who are members of the American Veterinary Medical Association have a good resource in the Career Development Center. The Center is divided into two parts: a job placement service, and individual counseling. You can get help via phone or mail, or by visiting the Career Center staff at their booth at any large veterinary meeting. Job openings are divided into practice and non-practice positions. There are usually a large number of practice positions listed.

The number of listings for non-practice jobs is relatively small, but still useful. The application form questions are extremely general, so don't worry about trying to focus on filling out the form in a way that targets a specific job. Leave your options open and you'll get a longer list of potential jobs. AVMA, 1931 N Meacham Rd Schaumburg IL 60173-4360; 800 248 2862; http://www.avma.org

Job search results

A recent application submitted to the Career Development Center for a non-practice job revealed this variety of job openings, none of which required more than a DVM degree:
- FDA position
- Veterinary technology teacher
- Extension veterinarian
- Consulting assistant (for veterinary business consulting service)
- Technical services rep for pharmaceutical company
- Sales rep for computer software companies (several different openings)
- Clinical trials coordinator for pharmaceutical company
- Primate facility veterinarian
- Pet food sales representative
- Food animal clinical researcher for pharmaceutical company
- Pork enterprise consultant

VETERINARY EXAMS AND LICENSURE

The new graduate with a DVM degree in hand must take and pass national and state exams in order to work in private practice.

The National Board Examination (NBE), a multiple-choice written test, is taken by senior veterinary students during or just after the senior year. Most states also require that DVMS take the Clinical Competency Test (CCT), another national written test that focuses on clinical skills.

Graduates of a non-US veterinary school must also obtain an ECFVG certificate (Educational Commission for Foreign Veterinary Graduates, run by the AVMA). The certificate requires credential verification, English language examination, passing the NBE and CCT, and passing a four day clinical practical examination (the Clinical Proficiency Examination) or completing a year of supervised clinical experience at a veterinary school.

By the year 2001 the NBE and CCT will be replaced by a single computerized, clinically-oriented, multiple choice test that will include graphic information such as photographs and radiographs. More sophisticated interactive computerized tests will be created in the future as finances permit.

Most states require that practicing DVMS have passed a state veterinary exam in addition to the national tests. Each state sets its own requirements for licensure, which may include an oral or practical exam in addition to a traditional multiple choice written test.

Some states offer the new graduate a temporary license before the test is taken. Others give the new grad who passes their test a temporary license for 6 to 12 months, and requires the new DVM to work under supervision during that time.

There is a trend for states to offer a "license by endorsement," which means that if the veterinarian is licensed in another state, has passed the NBE and CCT, and has practiced for a period of time (e.g., 3-5 years) without disciplinary action, then the board can issue a license by endorsement, requiring at most only a simple test over state rules and regulations. Over half the states have some type of license by endorsement or reciprocity now, and more are adopting it each year.

With regard to those states that don't offer license by endorsement, several state exams must be taken by veterinarians who are not sure where they may want to live or who think they may later move to another state. Another approach is to simply wait and see what happens to your career, and only take a different state's exam if you definitely want to move there. Once each state exam is taken and passed, you must pay a yearly fee for the privilege of retaining that license, or else suffer through re-taking the exam.

Some states require that you have passed the NBE within a period of three or five years of taking that state's exam; thus, a DVM who wants to move to another state, say, 10 years after graduation, may have to re-take the NBE in addition to taking that state's exam.

Because it becomes harder to pass tests after you've been out of school for many years, the best advice for recent graduates is to take tests in all the states in which you think you may want to practice, pay the fees for several years until you feel settled, then drop those licenses you are fairly sure you won't ever use.

Jobs that don't require licensure

DVMS who haven't passed the NBE, or those who have not taken or passed the state exam in a particular state, may still be eligible for certain non-practice jobs. Jobs that don't require passing the NBE may be found in government, industry, and academia.

Each state has its own definition of "practice"; that definition tells you which jobs require that the DVM has passed that state's exam. In general, veterinarians must have a license if they are serving the public for a fee. Exceptions may include consulting or research positions. Jobs that may require *a* state license, but not necessarily one in the state where the veterinarian is working, include many government and military positions, and some university positions.

Resources

1. *The American Association of Veterinary State Boards* publishes a directory of licensure requirements. Charlotte Ronan, Executive Director, PO Box 1702, Jefferson City MO 65102; 573-761-9937; aavsb1@socketis.net

2. *The AVMA Membership Directory and Resource Manual* (AVMA, 1931 N Meacham Rd, Schaumburg IL 60173) includes these resources:

• *The AVMA Model Veterinary Practice Act* lists common exceptions to the requirement for state licensure.

• *The Digest of Veterinary Practice Acts* includes requirements for practicing in each state.

THE LONG-RANGE OUTLOOK FOR THE VETERINARY PROFESSION

Continuing to believe in the stereotype of the "traditional veterinarian" as their *only* choice will lead many people to disillusionment and frustration. That point is well illustrated by an excerpt from Malcolm Getz' book, *Veterinary Medicine in Economic Transition.* Instead of letting this make you depressed, let it motivate you to take a strong look at *all* your options for greater long-term career success.

> "The market for veterinarians is already saturated. The supply of licensed practitioners has grown much faster than the demand for the last two decades to the point that career prospects are poor relative to other professions. The oversupply is likely to increase in the decade ahead as schools of veterinary medicine continue to produce many more veterinarians than the market can absorb. Career prospects will continue to deteriorate.
>
> "The superclinics may play an increasing role in the delivery of veterinary services, driving many small practices out of business and decreasing the demand for DVMs. In agriculture, corporate farming appears to be using fewer veterinarians more intensively. Careers in veterinary medicine are unlikely to become more attractive economically over the next decade."—*M. Getz*

The American Animal Hospital Association's *1995 Report* echoes that opinion: "There is excess capacity in the veterinary delivery system for companion animals...salaries for new and recent graduates remain very low (but) the majority have significant education debts to repay... Practice owners, on the other hand, are dealing with under-utilized facilities and an insufficient fee structure relative to the costs of providing services. Meanwhile, more practices are being opened, and veterinary colleges continue to graduate more and more small animal practitioners."

Many veterinarians *are* successful and happy working in private practice, of course; those people probably won't pick up this book. It's meant for the rest of you, and for those students astute enough to study their chosen profession before they make a blind entrance. Knowledge is power, and choices are the key to success.

Resources
Books
1. Veterinary Medicine in Economic Transition. Malcolm Getz, Iowa State University Press 1997.
2. Future Directions for Veterinary Medicine. William R. Pritchard. Duke University, Pew National Veterinary Education Program, 1989.
3. Veterinary demographic reports. Demographic and employment trend data. Center for Information Management, AVMA; 1931 N Meacham Rd #100, Schaumburg IL 60173
4. The 1995 AAHA Report. The American Animal Hospital Association, 1995.

Articles
1. Stagnant wages, increasing debt burden: Profession needs a plan. Kenneth Bovee. DVM Newsmagazine, 29(3) 3/97, pp 1 et seq
2. Is our profession prepared to address today's issues? P. Ray Glick. Veterinary Economics, 9/96, pp 34-38.
3. Reshaping the veterinary medical profession for the next century. N. Ole Nielsen. JAVMA 210(9) 5/1/97 pp 1272-1274.
4. Employment, starting salaries, and educational indebtedness of 1996 graduates of US veterinary medical colleges. B Gehrke. JAVMA 209(12) 12/15/96 pp 2022-2023. (Note: Similar report is published annually).

CHAPTER 2

PRACTICING VETERINARIANS' REQUIRED READING

This chapter is of particular value to practicing veterinarians who are thinking of changing their jobs, which usually means moving away from private practice. However, students should take note of this section, too—to get an idea of how veterinarians feel about changing their jobs. By anticipating that *this could happen to you,* you can avoid feeling that your life is ruined if your first job choice doesn't turn out exactly as you'd hoped.

Aren't I wasting my veterinary schooling if I'm not in practice?

One of the biggest stumbling blocks to avoid is the negative perception you may have about non-practice jobs. Others may say to you (or you may say to yourself), "Gee, won't you feel like you wasted your time in veterinary school, if you're not working in traditional practice?" I even had someone introduce me as "This is Carin Smith; she used to be a veterinarian." I had to explain that I still *am* a veterinarian—I just make a living in a different way than their dog doctor.

Have you ever thought to ask a small animal veterinarian, "Gee, don't you feel like you wasted your schooling? After all, you never use the bovine medicine, the herd health, the basic virology, or the histology that you learned!"?

Also consider this: You spent four years in veterinary school, with, at most, half of that in clinics—and half of clinics was spent working with species you probably don't see in your current job. Is it worth staying in a job where you're unhappy, just to prove that you "used" those years of your schooling?

Unfortunately, most people have a specific, romantic idea of what "being a veterinarian" is all about. You will encounter disappointment from people who feel you aren't fulfilling your (their) dream. It's also hard to have a job that people can't immediately visualize in a positive way. When you say you're a veterinarian, they immediately visualize a specific picture of a dog, cat, or horse doctor. When you say you're the director of technical services for a pharmaceutical company, or that you do medical writing, or that you work for the government, it's harder for others to imagine what you do.

Get ready for people to ask, "So, when are you going to go back to practice?" or, "Don't you miss working on puppies?" Prepare your animated, happy reply to "what do you do?," in a few sentences that include a brief description of what you actually do for a living. (e.g., "I'm a veterinarian, but like many veterinarians, I don't have a typical practice. Instead, my job involves .... . I really love my work!"

Another perspective on the "Aren't you wasting your schooling" thought: Aren't you wasting your time continuing to practice if it's not what you enjoy? What do you prove by staying in a job just because it's what you thought you wanted to do sometime in the past? How will you feel 5 years from now if you make a change, or if you don't?

Make a positive decision

For many veterinarians, thoughts of a change to non-traditional practice starts as dissatisfaction with their current jobs. However, to gain happiness in your new career path, you must be driven by more than the desire to get *away from* your old one. It's time to turn dissatisfaction into desire. This book can help you find a new career in veterinary medicine that you look forward to entering.

Enjoy your pursuit!

What about going back to school? (Don't I need another degree?)

The first option veterinarians tend to think of when considering careers beyond private practice is to go back to school—train in a different field, or specialize in a particular area of medicine or surgery. This is the method of change most publicized, and careers that require a DVM, plus another degree or board certification, are the ones that veterinarians know the most about. When reading about veterinary careers in just about any book, you find out that you can become a cardiologist, toxicologist, or laboratory animal specialist by going back to school. Or you may consider getting an MBA or law degree, and specializing in veterinary law or business.

The vast majority of veterinarians do *not* hold a degree beyond their DVM. About 6-7% of veterinarians are board-certified specialists; about 14% hold a Masters, PhD, or other advanced degree. If you're like most veterinarians, though, you probably don't have the desire, time or resources to go back to school. Perhaps you aren't sure enough of your potential new career choice that you are willing to commit to a few more years of school. What's more, getting a new degree (a new "career in a box") won't necessarily lead to greater happiness or success. Going back to school after all the expenses already incurred is sometimes not financially possible, nor will it always have a good impact on your personal life.

Finances are a real consideration for every DVM. The cost of veterinary school is high and the average debt upon graduation is staggering. Although returning to school means a longer delay before you can earn a decent income, board certification or pursuing a PhD *will*, on average, result in higher lifetime earnings. What's more, many student loans may be deferred until further training is completed.

The increase in income that results from further training is directly related to the type of work done. Advanced training yields far greater financial rewards for those who work in industry than for those who work at a university or for the government. The average income of someone with only a DVM degree who works in industry is higher than the average income of a board-certified DVM working for the government.

School isn't the only route to a new career. You have many more options for change than you may realize. And, you can get *started* in a new career without going back to school, to find out if you really like the change—then, later, you can always go back to school to further advance in your chosen new career (and sometimes, your employer will pay for it!).

Although this book focuses on jobs that do not require more than a DVM degree, that *doesn't* mean that all DVMs will qualify for all the jobs, nor does it mean that some kind of further experience or training aren't required. However, you should look beyond the traditional "going back to school and getting another degree" mentality, and see that your past degree(s) (BS or MS), work experience, seminars, internships, and independent study are acceptable ways to gain experience and become qualified for specific jobs. You can use your imagination and creative time-scheduling to create your own new learning situation. Don't immediately discount job ads that *appear* to ask for an advanced degree. During the research for this book, I encountered many people who said, "I didn't have the degree that's usually required for this job, but I got the job anyway, because of my special knowledge/talents/experience." Close inspection of job announcements often reveals statements such as "PhD *or equivalent research experience*," or "MBA *or equivalent business experience*." You might have just the specific experience they're looking for.

Resources

1. *Veterinary demographic reports*. Demographic and employment trend data, updated periodically. Center for Information Management, AVMA; 1931 N Meacham Rd #100, Schaumburg IL 60173

2. *Professional income of veterinarians employed by public or corporate organizations, evaluated on the basis of work experience, advanced academic degrees, and board-certification status, 1995*. JAVMA 210(8) 4/15/97 pp1112-1113.

3. *Marital disruption and higher education among women in the United States*. S. Houseknecht et al. Sociological Quarterly 21(3):375-389, 1980.

4. *Is advanced education worth the cost?* JAVMA 211(3) 8/1/97 Letter. C Smith & M Getz.

5. *The tenure trap*. John Davidson. Working Woman, 6/97.

Assess your skills and knowledge

The hardest thing about broadening your search for a new career is thinking of yourself in a new way. Rather than just "dog doctor" (or "horse doctor"), you have a compilation of skills and knowledge that is much broader than you think. Use your answers to the following questions to help beef up your resume.

1. What did you study as an undergraduate? Although you may have never officially "used" this knowledge or your BS degree, it is still a marketable attribute.

2. What were your jobs before you became a veterinarian? Did you help out in a research lab in college? Did you begin work on a Masters or PhD—even if you never finished? The skills you learned while doing that work should be listed on your resume. Many jobs in government and industry ask for knowledge of how to set up a research study or how to do research.

3. What kind of volunteer work do you do? What groups are you involved with? (Not just veterinary groups, but social groups, sports teams, Toastmasters, Rotary, parents' groups.) Have you ever been elected as an officer of any of those groups?

4. Have you ever written a scientific paper, a case study for a veterinary journal, a pet column for your local paper, or a newsletter for your clinic?

5. Have you ever spoken to your local Kiwanis group, or been interviewed by local television?

6. Have you taught 4-H classes, or community classes for adults?

7. What specific things have you done as a veterinarian? List your skills and areas of knowledge: radiology; anesthesia; surgery; pharmacology; toxicology; disease processes; medical terminology; ability to read and understand complex scientific reports.

8. What about administrative and managerial skills? How many employees have you supervised? What duties have you held in managing a veterinary clinic? Be specific, e.g., wrote budget, handled employee payroll, hired and fired employees, handled inventory.

Once you've broken down your experience into specific topics, you can see how diverse your knowledge and experiences are. Then you can start to see how your abilities can be applied to a wider variety of jobs than you'd ever dreamed. You may find that with some jobs the hiring agency may not be aware of the DVM's training and thus the job announcement won't be one you'd obviously target. For instance, a job with the United Nations titled "agricultural scientist" revealed, at closer inspection, the requirement for a "DVM or PhD in animal science." That job was not found simply by searching for "veterinarian."

Basic requirements for change

Specific qualifications needed for each job (besides holding a DVM degree) are listed in the discussion of the job itself. However, no matter what the job, whether in government or industry, at the AVMA or in technical writing, you must possess some basic skills and knowledge, which needn't be obtained via a college degree. What you need, in almost every case, are:

- Computer skills
- Oral communication skills
- Understanding of business
- Written communication skills
- Leadership and organizational ability
- A flexible attitude and a broad, diverse background

How are you going to get these skills? There are lots of ways to learn. Some cost money, yes—but think of this as "going back to school" in a whole new way. Consider how much less time and money this will consume, than would getting another degree!

Computer skills

- Get your own computer and software: word processing software; database software; *Internet access software.* Use it all. Play with it. Get comfortable with it. (You'll find that access to the Internet will greatly ease your job hunting, reduce your phone and mail costs, and save time.)
- Take classes given by your local school, adult education night classes, or correspondence/online schools.
- Subscribe to a computer magazine.
- Read books about how to use specific software.

Understanding of business

Practicing veterinary medicine helps you understand the private practice aspects of veterinary business; what about the rest? When you understand the business end of your potential career field, you are better able to tell your interviewers how your skills can enhance their company's goals. Studying can include reading (go to the library!), but also includes talking to people.

- If you want to write, you must understand the business of publishing (i.e., before a magazine will pay you to write an article, they want to know whether it's useful for their readers and subscribers).
- If you want to work in industry, you must understand their business.
- Go to veterinary meetings, visit the exhibit hall, and chat with the people there about what they do and what their company's goals are.

Oral communication skills

- Offer to give talks to local breeder's clubs, at veterinary luncheons, or for your local service organization. Keep a list of your speaking engagements for your resume.
- Join Toastmasters! I cannot recommend this highly enough. Through this club you can learn public speaking. Toastmasters has programs for all kinds of people to learn what they need most in their jobs. Look in your local newspaper for meeting times. Clubs generally meet before or after work hours, once or twice a month.
  PO Box 9052, Mission Viejo CA 92690; 800-9WESPEAK; tminfo@toastmasters.org   http://www.ni.net/toastmasters.org

Written communication skills

- Take a class in technical writing, magazine article writing, or other nonfiction writing given by your local school or online/correspondence courses.
- Write articles for your local breeder's club or saddle club newsletter.
- Write an article for a veterinary publication. (You needn't jump into publishing in refereed journals right away. Try *Veterinary Forum* or DVM *Newsmagazine* to start.)

Leadership and organizational ability

- Volunteer to be an officer in your local veterinary association or civic group.
- Help organize a veterinary meeting.

A flexible attitude and a broad, diverse background
You can't buy these attributes, but they're desired by most employers. Will you be able to change as a job changes, and as your employer's needs change? A diverse background is a plus in many jobs that require you to know a little bit about a variety of species, and to be knowledgeable about medicine, business, writing, and speaking. Employers know they can train you to do specific tasks if you are flexible and a good learner.

Essential skills

"The inability to drive a car in the old economy cut people off from a host of job opportunities. It's the same today with computers."—*Nuala Beck, in "Shifting Gears: Thriving in the New Economy." (Harper Collins 1992).*

How you can get further education, skills or knowledge
Use this list for general ideas. Specific educational opportunities may be listed in chapters discussing specific career paths.

Externships
These are not just for veterinary students! Ask whether you can spend a few weeks (or one day a week) working with someone for free, or at low pay—in exchange, you get to learn on the job, meet people, and find out what is involved in a career you may want to pursue.

Fellowships
The Federal Government and many universities offer paid fellowships for those who want to study in a specific area.

Home study / Distance learning
Courses on tape; correspondence or online courses; college courses via satellite TV.

Workshops and seminars
Attend meetings of the groups involved in your potential new career (Federal DVMs meeting, Extension agents' meetings, writers' seminars.)

Adult Education night classes
Through your community school or college.

Military training
Enlist part-time or full-time in the military and get free training in a variety of fields.

Study on your own
Subscribe to magazines and journals, and buy or borrow books about your area of interest. Read a book per week or per month, as your time allows.

Intensive learning courses
Many colleges offer short-term (weekend or 1-2 month) intensive courses in a variety of areas.

Volunteer
Do volunteer work for a nonprofit agency. Seek out an area where you need experience (writing, speaking, computer skills).

Resources

1. *College Degrees by Mail 1997: 100 Accredited schools that offer Bachelors, Masters, Doctorates, and law degrees by home study.* John and Mariah Bear, Ten Speed Press 1996
2. *Earn College Credit for What You Know.* Lois Lamdin, 1997
3. *The Oryx Guide to Distance Learning: A comprehensive listing of electronic and other media-assisted courses.* William E. Burgess, 1997
4. *College Degrees You Can Earn from Home.* Judith Frey, New Careers Center 1994
5. *The Electronic University : A Guide to Distance Learning.* Petersons Guides, 1993
6. *The MacMillan Guide to Correspondence Study.* Modoc Press Inc., 1996
7. *The Adult Learner's Guide to Alternative and External Degree Programs* (American Council on Education/Oryx Series on Higher Education) Eugene Sullivan, Oryx Press, 1993

Explore your limits

Self-assessment questionnaire
Are you thinking of leaving private practice? Before you zero in on a particular type of job, ask yourself some basic questions about your needs and your situation. The answers will narrow down your potential choices for a new career.

1. Am I (and is my family) able to move (to a different town in my state; to any other state; to another part of the world)?

Yes: Any career is open to you. If you *enjoy* travel, consider military or international assistance jobs.

No: Eliminate most government and corporate jobs, or be ready to take a job that might not be your first choice, simply because its location is right for you. Consider relief work, housecall practice, writing, consulting (involves travel, but you can live where you want).

2. Do I need a steady job with immediate good income and benefits? (To support a family, get good health insurance, pay off debt.)

No: Any career is open to you.

Yes: Eliminate housecall practice, relief work, writing, volunteer/assistance jobs, consulting. Consider a government job. If you want to get further training paid for, consider the commissioned corps or other military position.

3. Do I like working with people?

Yes: Most jobs are open to you. Focus on traditional private practice, teaching, consulting, industry's technical service, international assistance.

No: Consider writing, computer jobs, industry's research and development.

4. Do I like working as part of a team, or in a large group?

Yes: Consider corporate or government jobs, working with organizations or associations, or a job with an international assistance group.

No (prefer working alone, unsupervised): Consider relief practice, housecall practice, writing, independent contractor work for corporations (e.g., sales). Some animal care (AC) jobs with APHIS are fairly independent positions.

5. Do I need action and movement, or is a desk job preferable or acceptable?

Action: Consider traditional practice, relief or housecall practice; lower-level state jobs (advancement means moving to a desk job; lower levels involve the actual field work); APHIS veterinary service; FSIS (food inspector) jobs; sales jobs; R & D for industry.

Desk: Look at corporate management; Federal or state non-field positions; writing.

6. *Do I want regular hours, or am I able and willing to work odd hours or days? Would regular hours feel like a "rut?"*

Regular: Consider teaching, government, or military jobs.

Variety: Consider housecall or relief practice, writing, consulting, some corporate jobs. Food inspection can also involve long hours.

7. *Do I still want to work around or with animals?*

Yes: Consider traditional practice, housecall or relief practice; shelter work; industry, in research and development; teaching; or government, in veterinary services, APHIS.

No: Any job is open to you.

8. *Am I a new graduate, or do I have any private practice experience?*

No experience: Consider government jobs, or if looking at industry, be ready to start in an area that may not be your primary interest, just to get your foot in the door. Do not consider consulting, housecall or relief work until you have some experience.

Experienced: Any job may be open to you.

9. *Do I want to live in a city, or in a rural area?*

City: Most jobs are open to you.

Rural: Most states have DVMs working in "field offices" in various regions. APHIS field service jobs may also be located in rural areas. Consulting or technical writing can also be done from a rural home. Some industry jobs allow you to live in at least a small city, where you could find a home in the semi-rural suburbs. Extension agents often live in rural areas.

10. *Can I, or do I want to, work for someone else? If not, do I have what it takes to run my own business?*

Employee life is fine or preferred: Almost every career is open to you, except those listed next...

Self-employed is what I want: Consider technical writing, consulting, housecall practice, or relief practice.

11. *How do I feel about paperwork, policies, and regulations?*

That drives me nuts: Avoid working for associations, schools, the military, or government. Consider starting your own business (consulting, housecall, relief practice).

I can live with that: Associations, schools, the military or government jobs might suit you.

12. Make a list of the things you like and dislike about your current job.

Which of these will be different in your new chosen field? Which may be the same? Will a career change really bring you the changes you desire, or will it simply postpone your troubles, eventually leaving you with the same problems you have now?

Re-evaluate your limits

For many people, the primary restriction to life choices is that of geography. Because their family is living in one area, or their spouse has a job that can't be given up, their choices are restricted.

Others feel a need to continue to work with animals, or to help people. Let's go through the list of "I have to's" and see what comes up. Look for specific information about these choices in the chapters that follow.

1. I have to stay in my state. What are my best choices?

We can look to the AVMA's demographic data to find out which jobs are most abundant in your state. The following information is from 1995 data.

Approximately 1500 veterinarians are employed in veterinary industry. The numbers are highest in New Jersey, Pennsylvania, Michigan, Kansas, and California.

Approximately 700 veterinarians work for state or local governments. The greatest number are employed in Wisconsin, North Carolina, Florida, Texas, and California. However, every state employs a few veterinarians.

Military jobs are concentrated in Maryland, Texas, and US Possessions (e.g., Puerto Rico, Guam).

Civilian Federal jobs are concentrated in Maryland, Iowa, Texas, Georgia, and Virginia.

Jobs with the AVMA are in Schaumburg, IL and Washington, DC; jobs with AAHA, in Denver, CO.

Jobs you can create anywhere: housecall or relief practice; consulting; technical writing. APHIS jobs are located all over the country, too.

2. I want to work with small animals.

Consider working for APHIS in animal care; working for industry in research and development; or housecall or relief practice. Reminder: many government and industry jobs allow you to do relief work in private practice "on the side."

3. I want to work with horses, or horse owners.

Consider working for the APHIS in veterinary services; as an extension educator; or for industry, with companies that supply equine products or services. Reminder: many government and industry jobs allow you to do relief work in private practice "on the side."

4. I want to work with livestock, ranchers or farmers.

Consider working for a volunteer/assistance group in international positions, for the APHIS in veterinary services, as an extension educator, for the ARS (Agricultural Research Service), or for industry, with companies that supply livestock products or services.

5. I want to work with or help people directly.

Consider working for a volunteer/assistance program; working for industry, in technical services; working for the APHIS in veterinary services; international work; extension work; teaching; or working for the military. Also consider relief or housecall practice.

6. I want to work in another country.

Consider relief work, volunteer/assistance work, military jobs, or Federal jobs.

7. I'm not sure I really want to change jobs.

Ask for a leave of absence, and spend several weeks or months working with a volunteer or assistance group. Spend that time evaluating your life priorities. Or, look into short-term educational opportunities, externships, or short-term fellowships that allow you to explore a new field without making a long-term commitment.

8. Geeze, I'm stuck!

Are you placing so many limits on your job search that you have few choices left? If so, reconsider your "have to's."

Why can't you move to a different location? Can you move in order to begin your career change, with the potential of moving back to your desired area later on? Can you work as an employee until you gain enough experience to start your own business? Can you enjoy your pets and spend time with animals, even if a new career doesn't involve hands-on animal work? (Get any job with regular hours and good pay so you have time and energy to enjoy your own pets, train dogs, or ride your horse.) If you'd prefer an active job but can't find one, will the regular, predictable hours of a good-paying desk job allow you the time and energy to exercise (and money for club fees, ski vacations, and sports equipment)?

What are your priorities?

What trade-offs are you willing to make?

9. Is a job change really what I want?

If you find that you've placed too many restrictions on your "requirements for a perfect job," then maybe there isn't one. Are you dissatisfied with your job, or is your dissatisfaction with other aspects of your life? (i.e., are you searching for an answer in a new job, that cannot be found with a job change?)

Your search for the perfect job might result in the realization that the job you have now is the one that best fits your needs. That's great! Now you will feel less like complaining, and you'll dwell less on your problems. Instead you realize that your job is the one you'd choose out of all the choices in this book. You can now get on with it, making the best of your situation because you know you made a positive choice.

Another possibility is that you truly want to make a drastic change in your career. Perhaps you want to study art, accounting, or music. Such a dramatic change takes a lot of thought. A safe way to explore a new option is to study it part-time while continuing to work in the veterinary world part-time, thus keeping all your options open until you're sure enough to make the complete change.

Resources

1. *The Three Boxes of Life—and how to get out of them.* R. Bolles, 1978 (old but definitely *not* outdated!)
2. *What Color is Your Parachute?* Richard Bolles (several editions).
3. *Your Money or Your Life.* Joe Dominguez & Vicki Robin. Essential reading for those who feel they cannot make a change because they can't afford it. (Tells you *how* to do it!)

CHAPTER 3

TRADITIONAL VETERINARY PRACTICE

Your review of career choices in veterinary medicine begins with a discussion of traditional practice. What we mean by that term is the type of veterinary work that most people envision when they say the word "veterinarian."

PRIVATE PRACTICE

Small business

Traditional practice in its narrowest sense includes veterinarians who operate a small service business that provides health care for domestic animals owned by private citizens. "Health care" includes preventive medicine, anesthesia, surgery, diagnosis and treatment of disease, nutritional advice, emergency and intensive care, and all other aspects of medicine and surgery.

A *mixed practice* provides services for a variety of domesticated animals—including dogs, cats, horses, sheep, cattle, pigs, and goats. Many mixed-animal practitioners also work with "exotic" or "pocket" pets, which include ferrets, guinea pigs, reptiles, and birds. The mixed-animal practice is the typical practice in small towns and across rural America. Since these veterinarians are often the only ones available to the public in remote areas, they must be willing to work on all animals that are presented to their clinics.

The *small animal practice* (also called companion animal practice) typically is confined to dogs and cats. However, many small animal practitioners also work with birds, exotics, and pocket pets. Some DVMs concentrate only on exotics or birds, but this requires the large population base of a city. Large cities are also the primary location of *emergency clinics*—veterinary hospitals open only at night and on weekends. Trauma management and critical care are the focus of the emergency DVM's work.

Large animal practice can be divided into equine and food animal practice. Food animals include sheep, pigs, poultry, and cattle, but also ostriches and other exotic species. Some veterinarians work with all large animals, while others limit their practices to one or two species, or even to a specific type of animal within the species. For instance, within equine practice are veterinarians who may work only with race horses, show horses, or backyard "pleasure" horses; bovine practitioners may work only with dairy or beef cattle. Llamas are seen by equine or food animal practitioners.

The typical 4-year veterinary program offered at US veterinary schools emphasizes the above types of work. All veterinarians graduating from US veterinary schools will be prepared to enter private practice as described above, assuming they pass the board exams (see Chapter 1). However, what's often missed in this picture are these words: *veterinarians operate a small service business.* Veterinarians don't just practice medicine and surgery; they have to do all the work involved in running a small business—including supervising employees, marketing their business, and collecting payment from clients. Additionally, they spend a significant amount of time *working with people,* sometimes in difficult and emotional situations. Unfortunately, veterinary school offers them little or no preparation for those aspects of their work. DVMs must educate themselves about human psychology and business. Those who are successful (and who end up accepting their "real jobs," in contrast to the fantasy job we all, to some extent, envision as students), are the ones who enjoy their jobs. Others may find themselves reaching for other choices, including housecall or relief practice (see those chapters). Another alternative is to work in corporate practice.

Corporate veterinary practice

Although any practice may be run as an incorporated business, the term "corporate practice" has been used to describe a situation where several veterinary hospitals owned by one entity are run as a large business, often with branches in many cities. The words "corporate veterinary practice," "superstore," "superclinic," or "megapractice" have been used to describe these businesses. The emergence of corporate practices has many veterinarians frightened, and has caused an uproar within the profession, as is reflected by the headlines on every veterinary publication. Many veterinarians have strong negative feelings about corporate practice. We'll avoid passing judgement here, and just review some of the perceived pros and cons of large and small business operations.

Typically, the traditional veterinarian works alone or with several associate or partner DVMs. For some time, a hospital with 1-5 veterinarians was considered "typical." These veterinarians run their own business and deal with all the paperwork, administration, and decision-making that is required for running that business.

The basic approach of a corporate practice is to reduce costs and streamline procedures such that veterinarians can concentrate on practicing medicine and surgery and spend less time running the business. Corporate practices may own many hospitals in many states. These corporations may hire a large number of DVMs at a single hospital. That can save money when compared with the typical geographic area that has, perhaps, 10 different clinics, each with its own x-ray machine, surgical suite, and so on. Veterinarians employed by corporate practices may get superior pay and benefits compared with what they'd get in the average private practice (which often doesn't provide any benefits at all).

Corporate practices tend to create "policies," in an effort to avoid inconsistencies among the veterinarians' approaches. Whether or not that interferes with the individual DVM's ability to practice good medicine has been the object of considerable debate. Some argue that corporate practice reduces the potential for personal interaction between doctor and client or between doctor and staff members. Lack of control over business decisions may create conflicts for some veterinarians.

Many traditional veterinarians feel threatened by the corporate practices' ability to charge less for some procedures or products (which they are able to do because they can buy in volume and share resources). Corporate practices may offer a wider variety of products and services than do traditional veterinary hospitals. They may sell everything from dog toys to grooming aids. Some veterinarians view this approach as one that diminishes the professional aura of the veterinarian (after all, pediatricians don't sell children's toys); others insist that catering to every need of the pet owner is simply good business. Conflict-of-interest issues may arise between the need to sell a store's products and the provision of veterinary care, which sometimes offer incompatible services and products.

There are many shades of gray when you consider the types of practice that fall between the solo practitioner and the large corporate practice. Large urban practices may employ 5, 10, or 20 DVMs at one hospital. They may provide additional services, such as grooming and boarding, and they may sell pet products. They may hire a business manager such that the DVMs can spend more time being doctors and less time with business. Usually, some or all of the DVMs who work there are owners of the practice, and usually, they own only that practice. If they own more than one practice, it's usually in a nearby geographic area.

The issue of veterinarian ownership is a separate one from the issue of corporate versus small practice. A non-veterinarian or a veterinarian may own or co-own a practice of any size or one that is organized in any way. Practice owners may or may not work directly in, or manage, a practice that they own. And finally, state laws may allow or disallow non-veterinarian practice ownership.

The difference between veterinarians working in corporate practice and in traditional practice is one of business management, and is not a difference in careers per se. The

DVM in a small traditional practice will spend a significantly greater amount of time doing business management than will a DVM in a larger practice. Veterinarians interested in a career in traditional practice should examine their attitudes toward, and interest in, business when deciding where to look for jobs.

Species variety: fish to mink

Veterinarians may also decide to work with less traditional species, from fish and marine mammals to mink. One large area of interest is that of laboratory animal medicine. That includes mice and rats, but also larger animals up to the size of primates.

All veterinary colleges teach a bit about these species, but the student must usually make an extra effort to learn enough to create a career in that area (by spending extra time with the course instructor, by taking externships that involve that type of work, or by enrolling in an internship program after graduation). (An externship is a short-term work-study program required of all veterinary students.)

Veterinarians who work with poultry or mink are often hired to work full-time on large farms. Those who learn about marine mammals or fish diseases may be hired by government agencies (e.g., the Fish and Wildlife Service) or marine parks. Others focus on exotic animals and work in zoos. Laboratory animal veterinarians work in research facilities or universities and often go on to obtain further degrees (e.g., PhD) or board certification (see "specialists," below).

Alternative medicine

Some veterinarians want to stay in private practice (traditional *career*) and practice *alternative medicine*. The definition of alternative medicine changes over time, as formerly "alternative" practices blend into "mainstream" medicine. However, the term generally refers to areas such as veterinary chiropractic, homeopathy, and acupuncture. Veterinary colleges in the US teach little, if any, alternative medicine. Exceptions include the acupuncture courses taught at a few schools (e.g., U of PA, U of FL). For those who are interested, several groups offer information and courses for graduate veterinarians (see the current *AVMA Directory* for updated addresses; most of these groups use their current President's address for their contact point).

Resources
1. Alternative veterinary medicine online http://www.altvetmed.com
2. *American Veterinary Chiropractic Association*
Dr. Pedro Rivera
PO Box 249, Port Byron IL 62441
3. *Academy of Veterinary Homeopathy*
Dr. Jana Rygas
1283 Lincoln, Eugene OR 97401 503-342-7665
4. *American Holistic Veterinary Medical Association*
Dr. Carvel G. Tiekert
2214 Old Emmorton Rd, Bel Air MD 21015 410-569-0795
5. *International Veterinary Acupuncture Society*
Dr. Meredith Snader
2140 Conestoga Rd, Chester Springs PA 19425
or Dr. David Jaggar
268 West 3rd St Suite 4, Nederland Co 80466-2074

VETERINARY SPECIALISTS
Veterinarians in traditional practice may choose to specialize in one area of interest. Veterinary students get a good idea of the range of specialties within veterinary medicine while they are in school, because they are taught by many of these specialists. However, if you are not yet in veterinary school, you may not be aware of the potential areas in which veterinarians can specialize.

The word "specialist" has a legal definition. All veterinarians receive basic training in all of the areas listed here. Veterinarians in private practice who have only DVM degrees might do a lot of work in one area (e.g., surgery, behavior problems), but they are *not* considered "specialists." A veterinarian cannot be described as a specialist unless further training, beyond the DVM degree, has been obtained. Most specialties are organized within areas of medicine, not by species.

Veterinarians who want to specialize go through a postgraduate internship (usually one year) and then a residency (usually three years) in one area of interest. Their chances of being accepted for a program depend on their qualifications and on how flexible they are about where they will go. The internship or residency can be done at a university or a large private practice. Some are offered at places like zoos or marine parks, for those interested in wildlife or marine medicine. These are paid positions, but the pay is very low compared with that of the typical job in private practice. (Still, you're being paid to learn as well as to work.) Internships and residencies involve long hours or work and study, plus being on call for emergencies, with little time for anything else.

Veterinary specialties include:

Anesthesia
Behavior
Dentistry
Dermatology
Emergency and critical care
Epidemiology
Internal Medicine:
    Cardiology
    Oncology (cancer medicine)
    Neurology
    Internal Medicine
Laboratory animal medicine
Microbiology
Nutrition
Ophthalmology
Pathology
Pharmacology
Poultry medicine
Preventive medicine
Radiology
Surgery
Theriogenology (reproduction)
Toxicology
Zoological medicine

Following the residency, exams are taken to become "board-certified" in one of the specialties. There are currently about 5,600 board-certified specialists in the US; that's about 5-6% of all veterinarians. A board-certified veterinarian may find a job at a university, or in a large city in a private veterinary practice that employs several different specialists. Some are employed by veterinary industry, others by the government, and others work as consultants. The range of possible jobs for a board-certified veterinarian include all those discussed in this book; these people simply use different talents, they may be paid more, and they may achieve higher levels of promotion. (See Chapter 2: Going back to school.)

Board-certified veterinarians who stay in academia will find they aren't finished yet—they are strongly encouraged to pursue MS and PhD degrees in order to receive tenure (many DVMs choose to pursue a residency and a PhD or MS simultaneously). University work includes teaching veterinary students, conducting research, writing papers for publication in veterinary journals, and participating in committees, in addition to the hands-on animal work done in the specialist's area.

Resources

See also: Starting your own business; Housecall practice

Groups

See the *AVMA Membership Directory and Resource Manual* for current addresses of these and other interest groups:

American Association of Equine Practitioners
American Association of Bovine Practitioners
American Association of Feline Practitioners
American Association of Avian Practitioners
American Association of Zoo Veterinarians

Books

1. *The AVMA Membership Directory and Resource Manual.* AVMA, 1931 N Meacham Rd, Schaumburg IL 60196.
2. *Veterinary Ethics: Animal Welfare, Client Relations, Competition and Collegiality* Second Edition (chapter 16 discusses practice ownership and corporate practice). Jerrold Tannenbaum, Mosby-Year Book, 1995.
3. *Directory of Internships and Residencies.* Annual matching program. American Association of Veterinary Clinicians, 1024 Dublin Rd, Columbus OH 43215. 614-488-0617; Fax 614-488-0352.
4. *Veterinary Medicine in Economic Transition.* Malcolm Getz, 1997.
5. *Today's Veterinarian.* AVMA. 20-page booklet with a brief overview of careers in veterinary medicine, including list of colleges.
6. *Planning Your Veterinary Career.* American Animal Hospital Association, 1987; 1992. Out of print, but you may be able to find it through the library.

Articles

1. Professional income of veterinarians employed by public or corporate organizations, evaluated on the basis of work experience, advanced academic degrees, and board-certification status, 1995. JAVMA 210(8) 4/15/97, pp 1112-1113.

2. Is advanced training worth the cost? Letter. C. Smith & M. Getz. JAVMA 211(3) 8/1/97

3. Is an emergency practice for you? Thomas Catanzaro. DVM Newsmagazine 4/97 pp 9-15.

4. Survey of veterinary college curriculum requirements relevant to aquatic medicine. JAVMA 210(6) 3/15/97 pp 764-765. Analyzes whether veterinary schools really prepare students for this non-traditional practice. The same approach could be taken to analyze other types of work.

5. Employment, starting salaries, and educational indebtedness of 1996 graduates of US veterinary medical colleges. B Gehrke. JAVMA 209(12) 12/15/96 pp 2022-2023. (Similar report is published annually).

6. Veterinary Economics magazine, and *Veterinary Economics Reprint* Series (Includes: Marketing your practice; Charging fees with confidence; Starting a practice; and more). Veterinary Economics, 9073 Lenexa Dr, Lenexa KS 66215; 913-492-4300 ext 123.

7. Marital disruption and higher education among women in the United States. S. Houseknecht et al. Sociological Quarterly 21(3):375-389, 1980.

8. The tenure trap. John Davidson. Working Woman, 6/97.

CHAPTER 4

STARTING YOUR OWN BUSINESS

Many of the jobs described in the following sections *can* be performed by a veterinarian acting as an employee, but they usually are businesses run by one person who is self-employed. These jobs include consulting, writing, computer jobs, and housecall or relief practice (not to mention traditional veterinary practice).

Let's say you have come up with a great Widget that every veterinarian should buy for their practice, and you want to start a business selling Widgets. Or, you have written a great software program for veterinarians. Whether you are selling Widgets, software, or your housecall service, you must be proficient in two areas:

• You must know the technical aspects of your business (e.g., how to make a Widget, or how to use computers), and
• You must know how to run your own business.

The latter is just as important as the former. The biggest mistake made by new business owners is in thinking that their technical expertise will carry them through starting their business. Nothing will lead you to failure faster than that attitude.

SELF-ASSESSMENT QUESTIONNAIRE

Before you start your business, be honest with yourself about your abilities. Ask yourself:

- Are you interested in being your own boss, managing your time, disciplining yourself to work, selling your skills (or your Widget), and tracking down new clients?
- Are you good at record-keeping, or can you hire someone who is?
- Are you willing to study business management and make a business plan?
- What are your start-up costs? What equipment and supplies will you need? What ongoing costs can you project? What will you charge for your products or services?
- How will you target your market and analyze your competition?
- If your work involves travel, will you charge for travel time, travel costs, both, or neither?
- If you'll have an office in your home, is your area zoned for home offices?
- Do you have a good attorney and accountant who can advise you in legal and tax matters?
- Are you proficient at desktop publishing, so that you can create your own brochures, press releases, and other materials? (Your start-out budget often won't allow hiring someone for this!)
- Who are your potential customers, how will they pay for your product or services, and how will you handle late payments?
- Will you hire employees, and if so, to do what jobs?
- Do you have unrealistic expectations of the personal benefits of being self-employed? You may expect that you'll have more personal time, but chances are that you'll work longer hours than ever.
- What kind of insurance will you need?
- How will you pay your bills during the three to 12 months it will take to get your business off the ground?
- Can you get a loan to cover your business start-up costs?

Resources

See also: Traditional practice; Housecall practice; Relief work; Consulting; Jobs with computers.

Groups and Internet sites that offer free information and help

1. *The Small Business Administration* offers low-cost classes in starting a business, and a wide variety of publications that deal with every imaginable question you may have. Call your local chapter for more information, or write SBA Publications, PO Box 30, Denver, CO 80201-0030; 1-800-368-5855 or 1-800-827-5722. Their Web site has lots of great information, too! http://www.sba.gov

SBA publications include:

• Directory of Business Development Publications
• Checklist For Going Into Business
• Budgeting in a Small Service Firm
• Record Keeping in a Small Business
• Business Plan for Small Service Firms
• Profit Costing and Pricing for Services
• How To Get Started With a Small Business Computer

For the SBA's booklet, "Directory of State Small Business Programs," write to the Small Business Administration, Washington DC 20416. SBA loans are also available. The agency rarely loans money itself, but instead backs you with a loan guarantee at the bank. A group called SCORE *(Service Corp of Retired Executives)* can help you with free advice. Find the nearest group by contacting the SBA or Chamber of Commerce.

2. *The Edward Lowe Foundation* (ELF) provides information, research and education experiences which support small business people and the free enterprise system. The Foundation provides access to a vast amount of information through online services, computer databases, and publications written for small business people. The ELF Web site has a huge list of resources and links to Web sites for all sorts of other business information providers, including:

• smallbizNet is an informational clearinghouse for small business people; it includes the Edward Lowe Digital Library, a collection of approximately 4,000 full-text searchable documents (some free, some at a fee). Examples: OSHA handbook for small business; Starting and managing a business from your home.

• Entrepreneurial Edge Online is an electronic version of its print counterpart, providing practical advice and educational materials to aspiring entrepreneurs.

The Edward Lowe Foundation, 58220 Decatur Road, P.O. Box 8, Cassopolis, MI 49031-0008, 616-445-4200; http://www.lowe.org/

3. *The Small Business Resource Center* (Seaquest) provides online links to articles on starting and operating a small business, including: How to Prepare an Effective Business Plan; How to Raise Money to Start Your Own Business; The Legalities and Tax Advantages of a Home Business; How to Start a Consulting Service; Reorganize Your Time to Start a Home-Based Business. Seaquest also maintains a descriptive catalog of books and other media for small business owners.

seaquest@webcom.com http://www.webcom.com/seaquest
A list of free articles is found at
http://www.webcom.com/seaquest/sbrc/reports.html

4. *Smart Business Supersite* includes materials to help solve business problems, investigate industries, get trade show information, read about business news, and communicate with other small business owners. Most full-text material is free; a vast array of book titles and some newsletter subscriptions are available for purchase.
http://www.smartbiz.com   irv@smartbiz.com
5. *Small Business Law Center Forms and Model Documents* (some free, some for a fee). Automated drafting of documents for the computer industry, Internet commerce and general business transactions. Includes: How to Find a Lawyer; Links and Other Resources; Seminars and Discussion; Dealing with Lawyers - Some Helpful Hints; Business Organization; Intellectual Property; Legal Helpline; Legal Research Service. http://www.courttv.com/legalhelp/business/
6. *The US Business Advisor* gives information about government regulations, publications and resources for small business.
http://www.business.gov
7. *National Technological University.* Online short courses in business and other subjects. http://www.ntu.edu/
8. *Biz Resource* http://www.bizresource.com
9. *Business Forum* http://www.businessforum.com

Your state government:
Many states offer services or information for business owners. Contact the following agencies for information. Call information in your state capitol to get phone numbers. The names of these departments vary slightly from state to state.
1. The state department of taxation and revenue (economic development, board of revenue, etc): state taxes, business registration/licenses; some state departments have "new business owner" packets of information.
2. The state employment division (unemployment insurance, employment security, etc) for information about unemployment insurance
3. The state department of labor (labor and industries, worker's compensation department): worker's compensation coverage
4. The state veterinary board: licensing (accreditation is through USDA Veterinary Services)
5. The state licensing department: state business license, pharmacy or drug licenses

IRS Publications
Most libraries carry copies of all the following documents. If yours does not, write to the Superintendent of Documents, Government Printing Office, Washington DC 20402 or call 1 800 TAX FORM (800-829-3676) or get documents online at http://www.irs.ustreas.gov (All documents are free)

Handy IRS publications to review:
 # 553 Highlight of this year's tax changes
 # 334 Tax guide for small businesses

\# 463 Travel, entertainment, and gift expenses
\# 505 Tax Withholding and estimated tax
\# 533 Self-employment tax
\# 535 Business expenses
\# 552 Record keeping for individuals
\# 560 Self-employed retirement plans
\# 583 Taxpayers starting a business
\# 587 Business use of your home
\# 590 Individual retirement arrangements
\# 917 Business use of a car
\# 1200 List of IRS publications
\# 15 Circular E, Employer's tax guide
\# 937 Business reporting (Gives independent contractor criteria)
Form 1040-ES (Estimated tax for Individuals; includes explanation/worksheet)

Periodicals

Periodicals with information specific to a certain job are listed in the various chapters of this book. Those that are helpful for any job include:
1. *Home Office Computing.* Scholastic Inc., 730 Broadway, NY NY 10003. Excellent magazine directed at anyone with a home office.
2. *Tax Update for Business Owners.* 81 Montgomery St, Scarsdale NY 10583. Great tax tips; a must if you do your own taxes but also helpful for everyone to help keep tabs on the job your tax advisor is doing and to keep up with changes in the tax laws. Worth the steep subscription price.
3. *Entrepreneur.* 2392 Morse Ave., Irvine CA 92714
4. *PC World.* PO Box 55029, Bolder CO 80322-5029. Read for a better understanding of computers, and for product evaluations.
5. *In Business.* 2718 Dryden Dr., Madison WI 53704
6. *Success.* 342 Madison Ave., NY NY 10173
7. *Veterinary Economics* magazine, and *Veterinary Economics Reprint Series* (Includes: Marketing your practice; Charging fees with confidence; Starting a practice; and more). Contact Veterinary Economics, 9073 Lenexa Dr, Lenexa KS 66215; 913-492-4300 ext 123.
8. *Inc. magazine* PO Box 54129, Boulder CO 80322-4129; 800-234-0999; subscribe@incmag.com Great resource for the business owner.

Books

1. *Working from Home* (4th edition). Paul and Sarah Edwards. Tarcher/Putnam. Highly recommended! The classic book for any self-employed person with an office in the home—writers, housecall DVMS, relief DVMS, consultants, etc.
2. *Running a One-Person Business.* Claude Whitmyer. Ten Speed Press, 1989.
3. *How to Set Your Fees and Get Them.* Kate Kelly. Visibility Enterprises, 1986.
4. *The Joy of Working from Home.* Jeff Berner. Berrett-Koehler publishers.

5. *Successful Time Management: A Self-teaching Guide.* J. Ferner. John Wiley, 1980.
6. *Positively Outrageous Service: New & Easy Ways to Win Customers For Life.* T. Scott Gross. Mastermedia 1991.
7. *Your First Business Plan.* Joseph Covello. Sourcebooks 1993.
8. *How to Build a Successful One-person Business.* V. B. Bautista. Bookhaus publishing, 1995.
9. *Homemade Money: How to select, start, manage, market and multiply the profits of a business at home.* Barbara Brabec. Betterway Books 1994.
10. *The NAFE Guide to Starting Your Own Business.* Nat'l Assoc for Female Executives. (1-800-634-3966).
11. *How to Become Successfully Self-employed.* Brian R. Smith. Bob Adams Publishers, 1993.

Articles

1. *How to make a cash-flow projection.* Michael J. Strausser. Veterinary Economics, 5/93 pp36-46.
2. *Keep things separate to run a better business.* Linda Stern. Home Office Computing, 3/92 pp28-30.

CHAPTER 5

HOUSECALL PRACTICE

A housecall practice is a business where you go to pet (or horse) owners' homes to perform requested veterinary services. Most housecall practitioners keep offices in their homes, where they store client files, supplies and equipment.

The housecall practitioner comes in several varieties. The typical housecall veterinarian carries supplies in a vehicle, but performs work on pets in their homes. Some housecall veterinarians spend all their time on housecalls and refer any complicated cases to a full-service hospital; some may lease space in a clinic in which they perform in-hospital procedures (such as surgery) themselves; others work out of a "base" clinic and conduct housecalls only part of the time.

A mobile practitioner travels to the client's home, but performs work in a mobile "clinic," usually a form of motor home converted into an exam room, laboratory, and surgical suite. The large animal practitioner usually drives a pickup or large vehicle with refrigerator, running water, supplies and equipment in a self-contained unit such as those made by Bowie or LaBoit.

Both housecall and mobile practitioners can work part-time or full-time. They can work as employees or can be self-employed. A survey by the American Association of Housecall Veterinarians (AAHV) revealed that the "average" housecall DVM is a solo practitioner with no employees, whose business has been in existence for 5 years. This DVM drives an average of 20,000 miles per year, has 925 clients, works 50 hours per week, and has a cellular phone and an answering machine.

Daily work

Housecall veterinarians focus on preventive medicine and minor procedures that don't require hospital equipment or staff. They see fewer clients per day than does a veterinarian in a hospital, for two reasons: first, much of their time is spent driving; and second, they spend more time with each client. Housecall DVMs may develop a more personal relationship with their clients than do other veterinarians. They may perform more euthanasias than the average DVM, because even people who ordinarily take their pets to a veterinary hospital will call upon a housecall DVM for this service. Housecall DVMs also may focus on behavioral problems in pets, since solving these problems is easier when the home environment can be evaluated.

During a typical day, the housecall DVM will see 10 clients and will spend quite a bit of time driving. The job requires self-sufficiency and self-confidence, since there is no one to provide help or advice during the day. These veterinarians become adept at drawing blood from a cat without restraint, using a cellular telephone, helping clients deal with grief after euthanasia, and organizing their driving schedule to minimize time-consuming backtracking. Those who are able to work with birds and exotic animals as well as cats and dogs will have an advantage, since the former pets are difficult to transport to a veterinary clinic.

Pros and cons

A housecall practice allows you to set your own schedule and hours. That allows you to work around your clients' schedules more effectively, too. Professional benefits include working in a challenging environment that changes every day, working alone without employees, and owning your own practice with low overhead costs. You can also develop a more personable relationship with your clients; create a more leisurely schedule; and enjoy the calmer behavior of animals not stressed by a car ride or clinic atmosphere. You may be able to assist those who are unable to transport pets to a clinic, or who cannot leave the home; evaluate the effect of a pet's environment on its health; and get more done at your own home, since you aren't stuck sitting around at a workplace when there's no work to do.

Some disadvantages to consider:
• You may have difficulty separating your work and personal life.
• You are dependent on a vehicle that runs well.
• You may miss the camaraderie of working with other veterinarians.
• You can't perform much surgery.
• Clients who are friends may tend to assume you are always available, or that you'll give them discounts.
• Your liability may be higher because you often have pet owners assist you (a main cause of lawsuits is injury to pet owners who restrain their own animals).
• You have to put up with driving and traffic.
• You have less assistance than you would in a hospital.
• Because of the increased client interaction time, plus travel time, fewer clients can be seen per day.
• You aren't building up equity in something you can later sell, as you would with a normal clinic. Since it is hard to sell good will and a client list, you must be careful to sock away sufficient retirement funds.
• You have all the administrative responsibilities of a business owner.

Pay

Housecall veterinarians can earn as much as most traditional-practice veterinarians. Although it is not possible to see as many clients in a day as you would in a typical clinic, that's balanced by your reduced overhead expenses and the higher fee you charge for each visit. There are limits, though, when comparing a practice owner with a housecall DVM. The practice owner receives not only current income, but also (theoretically) a return on the investment in land, a building, and a client base.

Fees charged by housecall DVMs will parallel those charged by clinics and hospitals in the area, with the addition of a "housecall fee" that is charged over and above the exam fee.

Qualifications

The housecall practitioner is the chief executive, the main employee, and in many cases, the bookkeeper, technician, receptionist, and veterinarian all rolled into one. Since the housecall DVM has an office in the home, the local zoning code must allow for home-based businesses, and there must be space for an office in the home. Successful housecall DVMs are comfortable working with people on a one-to-one, friendly basis, and are outgoing, personable, and self-assured. They have the self-discipline necessary to organize their working hours, manage their business, and schedule non-work time. They have enough experience to handle, by themselves, any situation that might arise. Housecall veterinarians know that if their abilities or the home environment are inadequate to perform a particular treatment, they will have to refer that patient, and they must give up performing certain procedures that are best done in a hospital.

Veterinarians who might *not* like housecall work include those who prefer having a qualified technician's assistance, or who thrive on the exchange of ideas and information among veterinarians in a group practice. Veterinarians will be most successful with housecall practice if they have at least a year or more of practice experience. Those who are comfortable chatting with other DVMs online via computer will minimize their professional isolation.

One approach to starting a housecall practice is to continue at your current job and set up your house call practice as a separate business that you work on during your "off" time (with your present employer's agreement), and leave your regular job after a designated time period. Another approach is to work part-time (a few days a week, or a few hours a day) at a veterinary clinic to keep some income, and start your housecall practice part-time.

Some DVMs choose to work as relief veterinarians while they begin housecall practice. This will be difficult. Most relief jobs last a week, and you won't be able to see any of your new clients during this time; if your "relief" job consists of working specific days of the week or specific hours each day, then you are a part-time employee—not a relief veterinarian.

Some veterinarians find that they can integrate housecalls into their current jobs, continuing as an employee or partner in the practice. Finally, one choice is to save up money, get a loan, or rely on your spouse's income while you start a full-time housecall practice right from the beginning.

Resources

See also: Starting your own business.

Groups

American Association of Housecall Veterinarians is a loosely organized group that sporadically publishes a newsletter and meets during the annual AVMA meeting and other conventions. See the current *AVMA Directory* under "Associations," or look for a meeting notice on the bulletin board at any large veterinary meeting.

Results of a 1992 survey of housecall DVMs can be obtained from Dr. Stan Glass (At Home Veterinary Care, 7401 SW 84th Pl, Miami FL 33143), or by contacting the AAHV (see above)—the survey results were published in their January 1993 newsletter (Vol 4, No. 1). (The survey includes type of vehicle used, practice name, length of time in practice, number of employees, hours worked, services provided, fees charged, and more.)

Books

The Housecall Veterinarian's Manual. Updated periodically. This workbook includes detailed information about setting up your home office, creating an agreement with a local veterinary hospital for in-hospital work, setting your schedule, getting clients, setting fees, hiring employees, and more. Smith Veterinary Services, 1997. PO Box 254, Leavenworth WA 98826; 509-763-2052; smithvet@nwinternet.com http://www.now2000.com/smithvet

Articles

1. *Ready for house calls?* Carin A. Smith, DVM. Veterinary Economics 2-part series, 2/97 pp 62-68; 3/97 pp 90-95.
2. *Career Paths: Housecall practice.* Perspectives May/June 94 pp 60-65.
3. *The happiness and headaches of house-call practice.* M. Major. Veterinary Economics 12/91 pp 61-64.
4. *Practice shines, thanks to Millie.* R. Dahlem. Veterinary Economics 9/94 pp 68-69. (receptionist for mobile practice).
5. *Options for a housecall practitioner who wants to sell his client records.* Veterinary Economics, 6/95 pp 20.
6. *What's an equitable leasing arrangement for a surgical suite?* Veterinary Economics, 9/94, pp 21.

7. *Financial arrangements when a specialist rents space in your practice.*
(Practice Management Q & A). Veterinary Economics 8/95 pp 24.
(Although this refers to a specialist, the basic concept of renting practice
space is the same).

8. *Leasing your practice to another veterinarian?* (Practice Management Q
& A) Veterinary Economics 9/95 pp 22.

9. *Trust examines insurance needs for a house call practice.* P. Stilts.
JAVMA 205(3) 8/1/94 pp 397-8.

10. *Scope out your colleagues' fees!* Nationwide fees report. Veterinary
Economics, 10/95, pp 30-38.

CHAPTER 6

RELIEF VETERINARIAN

A relief veterinarian is someone who makes a living working a series of temporary jobs (or "locum tenens"). The relief veterinarian offers services to other veterinarians for a short-term, temporary "relief" situation. Each job may last as short as a half day or as long as several weeks. The reliever can take enough jobs to work full-time, or can work only part-time, as desired.

Daily work

The relief DVM keeps a small home office from which jobs are scheduled and paperwork is completed. A typical month might include working a week at a nearby small animal clinic; working a weekend at an emergency clinic; and traveling to a nearby small town to work at a mixed practice, staying in a hotel or in the absent veterinarian's vacant home. These small-town jobs usually include taking emergency calls during the night.

Relievers do not work regularly at any one clinic. If a DVM works every Monday for Dr. Jones, for example, then that DVM is a part-time employee, not a relief veterinarian. However, relievers can and do work more than once for any one hospital—for example, the reliever could cover for Dr. Jones during several veterinary meetings, holidays, and vacations scattered over a year's time.

Relief DVMs respond to calls from interested veterinarians by first confirming they are available on the requested dates. Then the reliever states his or her fees, and the caller decides whether or not to hire the reliever. The reliever sends a contract or letter that confirms the verbal agreement.

Once on the job, the reliever sees appointments, performs surgery, and cares for animals in the hospital. Relievers are legally and medically responsible for any cases in the hospital where they are working, so it is important that they agree with the philosophy and medical standards of the hospital owner. Relievers walk the tight rope of trying to maintain the clinic's "standard" policies and procedures, but maintaining their own standards of practice at the same time.

The amount of travel required for a relief DVM depends on the type of work done and the size of the community. Relief DVMs who live in a large city and limit themselves to small animal work may not need to travel at all. However, those who live in a smaller town may need to travel extensively to get enough work to keep busy full-time.

Relievers who have an unusual talent may also travel more, since hospitals that need those special services are less likely to find someone in their own geographic area. Thus relievers who are willing to work on large animals, exotics, or birds may find that their services are requested over a wide geographic area.

Working on weekends, holidays, and during popular continuing education meetings is assumed by relievers. They plan their vacations at times when others typically don't take theirs, are ready to celebrate holidays on the day before or after the actual date, and plan their CE around other DVM's preferences. Relievers will get more work if they are willing to take emergency calls. However, doing so means working after hours, perhaps more than veterinarians employed in a regular job.

Pros and cons

Many of the advantages of relief work are similar to those of housecall practice. This career allows for great flexibility and control over personal time and income. The reliever who does a good job and is willing to travel (or who lives in a large city) will have no shortage of work. Disadvantages include travel and working on holidays and weekends. Relievers often have to go to less popular or out-of-area continuing education meetings, since they'll likely have relief jobs during local meetings. Relievers must work with new people all the time—some they may like, and some not. The reliever has little control over the clinic atmosphere and policies, and can't easily follow up on cases.

Pay

The fees charged by relief veterinarians vary according to the local economy. Fees may be charged by the hour or by the day. Most relievers charge a base hourly fee, with a minimum daily fee. Typical fees in 1997 range from $200-$400 per day, or $30-50/hour. Additional fees are charged for mileage to any clinic out of the area; for use of any of their own equipment; for hotels; and for taking emergency calls.

Over the long term, relief work can provide a satisfying full-time or part-time career. Relief veterinarians sometimes work back-to-back shifts (day clinic/emergency clinic) in order to earn money quickly in the short term (for paying off loans or returning to school).

Relief DVMs must realize that because they do not own a practice, they aren't building up equity in something that will pay them back in retirement. Thus, the career relief DVM must take extra care to sock away money for retirement.

Qualifications

Consider the following questions when considering whether you'd like relief work:

• Are you interested in operating your own business and being self-employed?
• Are you comfortable working with people with a variety of personalities? Are you outgoing, personable, and self-assured?
• Are you able to work alone, or are you accustomed to a qualified technician's assistance? Do you have enough experience to handle any situation that might arise when you are

the only veterinarian? Relief work is not always a good job for new graduates; the kinds of experiences gained when you are left alone are not necessarily good ones. You must be confident and decisive working on your own.

• Are you comfortable with any and all anesthetic regimens? Are you able to use a variety of methods, medications, and equipment, or do you prefer one set protocol? Are you comfortable looking up information as needed?

• Are you able and willing to travel? Can you work on holidays and weekends? Are you flexible enough to work different hours each week? Can you take your own vacations at odd times of the year?

• Are you meticulous with record-keeping? Do you write every detail in the patient records?

• Can you write up charges at each clinic according to their policies, or are you accustomed to altering your fees as you see fit for each case?

• If your facilities are inadequate to perform a particular treatment or surgery, are you comfortable with referring that patient (even though you have the expertise to take care of the problem)?

• Are you able to maintain your high standards of practice in spite of your surroundings?

• Are you ready to turn down jobs in clinics where you are not comfortable, even though you need the work? If you take such jobs, are you ready to assume the liability for all cases handled there?

To start

Many people start doing relief work quite casually. However, to take the full tax advantages of being self-employed, you should go to the trouble of setting up a genuine business. Start by estimating your expenses and establishing your fees and policies. Get a business license (not the same as the veterinary license) and write up a contract for every job. Make a plan for marketing your services. Be sure you have enough savings to carry you through your initial slow time.

Relief veterinarians are self-employed (that is, they are independent contractors); they are not the employees of the clinics where they work. They have their own business licenses, set their own fees and policies, work for a specified number of days, and then collect their fee after giving the hiring DVM or hospital a bill. They are not paid on a regular pay day. They do not have a continuing relationship with any one hospital, although they may be hired more than once by one clinic. They cannot be fired since they are hired only for a specific period. Thereafter, they may be hired again or not hired again, and they may accept or turn down any future job offers.

It is essential that relief veterinary service is distinguished from the job of a part-time veterinarian. A part-time DVM is an employee who works a specified number of hours or days at one clinic (consistency is the key, not the number of hours worked). For instance, if you work from 9 to 12 every Monday for Dr. Jones, you are considered a part-time employee at that practice. You receive a regular pay check on regular pay days.

If you are a true relief DVM, then you can take certain tax deductions that are allowed for self-employed people. If you are a part-time employee, you should receive benefits that are given to all employees. If you mis-classify yourself, then you and the person hiring you may be subject to penalties in the event of an audit.

Agencies

Many relief veterinarian agencies are springing up across the country. Their services vary from simple matching of relief DVMS and job requests, to more advanced services that include screening of both the job site and the relief DVM. Very few agencies offer enough benefits to outweigh their downside—a restrictive covenant and potentially lower fees than you'd make on your own. However, at least one agency has modeled itself after those for human physicians, and hires relief DVMS as full-time employees, placing them in a variety of jobs in the midwest. (Because of the way their business is set up, this is one situation where relief DVMS are classified as employees—but of the *agency*, not of the clinics where they work.)

Resources

See also: International jobs—relief work; Starting your own business.

Groups

1. The Veterinary Independent Contractors Association
(Has newsletter, "Vet Web"; meets at various national conferences).
1 Argonaut #250, Aliso Viejo CA 92656; 714-457-8810; Terry Honer,
DVM, 1659 N Refugio Rd, Santa Ynez CA, 93460-9312; 500-437-8617;
dvm relief@aol.com
2. Midwestern Veterinary Relief Service (agency). PO Box 56, Westerville,
OH 43086; 614-337-1888.
3. For *worldwide relief openings*, contact: Envirovet Ltd Ivy Wood,
Westrop Green, Cold Ash, Thatcham, Berkshire RG18 9NW, England.
UK Voice: +44-1635-202886 Fax: +44-1635-202886
vetlocums@envirovet.demon.co.uk   http://www.vetlocums.com/
4. Your state or local veterinary association:
The San Diego County (CA) Veterinary Medical Association has done
extensive research on independent contractors, accumulating a wealth
of information, legal documents, case studies, and other information
that affects independent contractor relief veterinarians. The Washington
State Veterinary Medical Association has worked with the state
department of labor and industries, and the employment security
department, to define the status of relief veterinarians. An explanatory
article is available from the WSVMA.

Books

1. The Relief Veterinarian's Manual. (updated every two years). Includes
details about how to set fees, how to get work, tax tips, and more—
including sample contracts. Smith Veterinary Services, PO Box 254,
Leavenworth WA 98826. 509-763-2052; smithvet@nwinternet.com
http://www.now2000.com/smithvet
*2. The Employer's Manual: A Guide to Hiring Part-Time and Relief
Veterinarians.* Includes guidelines for creating contracts for part-time
veterinarians. Carin A. Smith DVM, Smith Veterinary Services 1993/
1997.

Articles

1. The Business of Being a Relief Veterinarian. Carin Smith. Veterinary
Economics, 12/90 pp 62-67.
*2. Trust, Respect, Competence Lead List of Qualifications for Relief
Veterinarians.* C. Smith. DVM Newsmagazine, 7/88 pp 50 et seq
3. Good Communication Key to Relationship with Relief Veterinarian. C.
Smith. DVM Newsmagazine, 10/91 pp 52 et seq
4. Plan for Relief Help to Take Surprises out of Hiring Decision. C. Smith
DVM Newsmagazine 11/91 pp 24 et seq
*5. Clear Communication with Relief DVM Essential to Avoid False
Expectations.* C. Smith. DVM Newsmagazine 12/91 pp 26 et seq
6. Which is it? Independent Contractor or Employee? by Owen McCafferty,
CPA Veterinary Economics, 5/90, pp 74-79.
*7. Employed Veterinarians as Independent Contractors—Some Legal
Considerations* H. W. Hannah, JAVMA 9/1/87 pp 502-503.

8. *Need More Flexibility in Your Life? Try Relief Work.* Julie Hoenisch. Perspectives Mar/Apr '96 pp 31-37.
9. *Relief veterinarian.* Diane D'Orazio. JAVMA 197(3) 8/1/90 pp 340-341. (Includes some incorrect information about relief DVMs that actually applies to part-time employees, but otherwise good).

CHAPTER 7

CONSULTING

A consultant is someone who charges a fee to share special knowledge and to give specific help or advice to a client. The advice can be in the area of business, medicine, computers, livestock management, or just about anything else. Veterinarians can work as consultants for businesses ranging from veterinary clinics to livestock feed companies. For instance, one veterinarian with an extensive background in animal shelter work is hired by shelters to train their employees. Another works as an international consultant, traveling all over the world to gather and disseminate information about new breeds of pigs.

Consultants are hired for assistance in a specific problem area (which can be broad or narrow) for a specified length of time (which can range from weeks to years). A consultant is a combination of teacher, leader, and mentor who leaves each client with solutions and new ideas that can be put into practice long after the consultant has gone.

Daily work

Consultants can work on their own or as part of a team. They usually travel frequently, since they are most effective when they have seen and evaluated their clients' environment.

Personal visits are preceded by background study, and are followed by telephone consultations. Before an on-site visit, the consultant obtains as much information as possible about the client to maximize time efficiency during the visit. The consultant's office work may include studying demographics; writing materials such as office manuals, contracts, and client educational materials; analyzing financial, medical, or nutritional data; writing articles and speeches; developing ideas for seminars, then marketing and planning the specifics for those seminars; and keeping up with reading in the consultant's area of expertise.

Veterinarian-consultants may be hired by

Other veterinarians
Livestock producers
Livestock feed companies
Farm equipment companies
Veterinary medical equipment companies
Veterinary computer software companies
Pharmaceutical companies
Attorneys

The consultant working solo has a small office that may be kept in the home. This work space requires a computer, telephone, answering machine, and fax machine. A cellular phone helps the consultant keep in touch with clients while on the road.

Consultants frequently use computer programs to analyze data, to communicate with clients via electronic mail, and to keep their own records. Consultants have to market their own business, too, which is done by word of mouth and advertising, including creating advertisements or announcements for direct mail solicitation or for use on the Internet. They also attend meetings that are likely to be attended by their potential clients, to meet people and spread the word about their services (veterinary, producer, equipment, and feed company trade shows).

Most consultants are regular speakers at veterinary and related industry meetings. Speaking is a way to educate as well as to let potential clients evaluate the consultant's expertise. Many consultants also create their own seminars, which they offer independently from other veterinary meetings. Clients may attend these seminars as a way to pick up business tips, and then decide to hire the consultant for specific help.

Consultants also publish regularly in journals or magazines appropriate to their area of expertise (e.g., business consultants might write for *Veterinary Economics* magazine; livestock consultants write for livestock publications). Writing is done for the exposure, to disseminate word about their work, to establish their credentials, and to educate potential clients about the benefits or need for their services.

Pros and cons

Consultants are problem-solvers who make a living helping people do things better, faster, cheaper, and easier. Consultants must travel frequently, be comfortable speaking, stay cheerful and positive with every client, be flexible, and enjoy working with and helping a wide variety of people. They spend a lot of time on the telephone. Consultants are team leaders. Writing skills are necessary and are often used (all verbal recommendations must be followed up in writing; consultants often produce newsletters for their clients). Consultants must continuously come up with new solutions for new problems, easily changing their approach for different clients. Consultants can be self-employed or work for a company; they may work alone or in a group.

The consultant often causes clients to be initially dissatisfied—by pointing out problems, and by making changes, which no one likes—before they are satisfied. The consultant must differentiate between what their clients want and what they need. Consultants may carry a large accounts receivable, so collecting payment is a constant job. Soliciting new clients is an everyday need (direct mail, attending meetings potential clients might attend, speaking, etc). Some clients may become "management junkies," who revolve through a series of consultants without making any positive changes. Such clients can be frustrating to work with. Other clients don't take the advice given and thus don't see any benefit.

Livestock consultants may depend on a small number of large corporate clients, creating a risky business situation if one client is lost. Livestock consultants also may find that their *business* advice is not solicited or followed because they are viewed as being experts in *medicine* only.

Consultants need to be able to put a dollar benefit value on the advice they give. That is, they must be able to show with numbers that their fee will be recouped in higher profits for the client.

Swine consultant

"I work for a private company that is implementing a bilateral (Chinese-Canadian) livestock development project for the Canadian International Development Agency (similar to AID in the US). As the project veterinarian, I am responsible for the health of three project swine herds located in China. I live at one site, where I'm the site manager, and visit the others on a quarterly basis.

"The job can be very challenging—it can be difficult to find some animal health supplies, such as biologicals and pharmaceuticals, and we have had to create our own diagnostic support system for the farms. My daily work involves a lot of training and interaction with my Chinese colleagues. This may take the form of discussions and hands-on demonstrations, or, occasionally, more formal lectures. I also assist with technical problems. I enjoy problem-solving at the farms and seeing people use knowledge that they have acquired as a result of the project."

—*Janet E. Alsop*, DVM, *China-Canada Lean Swine Project, Yutian, Hebei Province, PR China*

Consultants who work alone may work long hours and get little time off. Their businesses consist of blue sky (no product, just a service) based solely on their own work. It may be difficult to build up equity and create a saleable business—thus they may have nothing to show at retirement. Like other self-employed people, they must concentrate on creating a good retirement fund. Hiring another DVM with the goal of selling the business to him or her is a good idea.

Pay

Consultants charge $100 per hour and up, a daily fee (up to $3000 per day), or an annual fee with monthly payments (common with livestock consultants, who may be hired long term). More is charged for giving seminars. Hourly fees may be broken down into increments (1 minute, 15 min, etc.), and variations of fee structure are common (e.g., fee per month, fee for basic job plus hourly fee on top). Remember that not all work time is billable time. Marketing, office recordkeeping, studying (when not for a specific client), preparing speeches, and some travel are done on your own time and at your own cost. Clients tend to prefer a basic fee with "extras" built in, rather than to see a bill with all kinds of little charges added for phone, copying, etc. (One expert advises that veterinary businesses hiring a consultant should not spend in excess of 1% of their hospital's annual gross income.)

Management consultants may work for a client on a short-term basis (a few days, weeks or months); they may be hired for a year at a time, to help with long-range projects; or they may be hired for repeated management services, helping with bookkeeping, accounting, or human resource management.

Qualifications

Consultants must have a great deal more experience and breadth of knowledge than do their clients. However, specific skills are required in addition to their technical knowledge. Consultants must also have top-quality writing and speaking skills, and they must be great communicators, able to interact with all kinds of personalities. They must be knowledgeable about human behavior, needs, and desires, and be effective at motivating people to work together as a team. They must understand the fear of change and how to help their clients overcome that fear with positive results. Computer skills are essential (at a minimum, the ability to use a variety of software programs and online services; at a higher level, the ability to tailor specific software to a client's needs). Many consultants get additional business training to aid in the business aspects of consulting. Consultants must be comfortable leading, working alone, selling their skills, and tracking down new clients.

A consultant's expertise can be gained through previous work experience. One way to gather more experience in your path to consulting work is to take a job with the government or in industry. That way you get paid for your time and you learn on the way. Take the opportunity to work in a variety of career paths, even those you don't like, in order to broaden your background and knowledge. See the sections on government, industry, volunteer, and association work for more details.

Another route to expertise is by taking classes or gaining advanced degrees (in business, finance, livestock management, economics, healthcare administration, or agribusiness). You needn't worry about leaving your job and "going back to school." More and more universities are offering short-term intensive courses, or correspondence or online courses. Others have branch programs targeted at working people. You can take courses with or without the intention of getting a degree.

TYPES OF CONSULTING

Business consultant

Business consultants evaluate the internal operations of a veterinary clinic or other business and assist the owners in areas of weakness. They work with business owners or managers to improve the performance, profitability, and goals of the company.

Assistance may be offered in:
• Using staff effectively
• Evaluating staff pay and benefits
• Effective time management
• Ensuring compliance with OSHA regulations
• Improving competence of doctors (in medicine or surgery) or staff (technical or receptionist duties)
• Development of a new practice

- Moving to a new location, or planning a new facility
- Improving paperwork (medical records, contracts, hospital manual)
- Targeting new clients
- Monitoring income and expenses
- Preparing a marketing plan
- Reducing taxes, using proper tax forms, or keeping up with changes in tax law
- Installing, updating, or improving the use of computer and software
- Creating custom software for the business
- Assisting with partnership negotiations or practice sales
- Planning for the future

Livestock consultant

A *livestock consultant* evaluates all aspects of a livestock production facility to increase profitability. Although many producers take care of their own vaccinations and treatments for common diseases, this practice may actually increase their need for a consultant. The veterinarian can advise the producer about which vaccines are most cost-effective and which antibiotics are appropriate for particular situations.

The veterinary consultant gives recommendations about:
- Management
- Medical care
- Preventive medicine (e.g., which vaccinations and dewormers are cost effective to use?)
- Nutrition (balancing or analyzing rations, finding less costly feed ingredients, analyzing use of supplements)
- Genetic counseling and evaluation of breeding lines
- Facilities/housing (size, number of animals per unit of space, cleaning procedures, sanitation, potential for disease transmission, ventilation)
- Computer programming
- Interpretation of data generated by a computer program
- Defining a corporate mission, market segments, and market potential for a client
- Evaluating pricing, promotion, distribution, and sales
- Training staff
- Keeping up to date with new technical developments and information

Livestock consultants usually start by working with individual clients (farmers/ranchers). They can then choose to continue to work with larger numbers of individuals, or to work for larger companies. Work for companies can be done as an employee or on a freelance basis. The consultant must be aware of and in contact with experts in related fields, such as nutritionists and geneticists, to make use of their expertise when appropriate. Sometimes several experts work together in one consulting firm (with the DVM as overall manager) to provide all necessary services to each client.

Livestock consultants have an opportunity for international work. For instance, one swine practitioner is involved in a Canadian-Chinese livestock development project. This DVM is responsible for herd health, staff training, and problem-solving for swine herds at three sites in China.

Industry consultant

An industry consultant assists companies by:
- Tracing the source of poor product performance in the field
- Evaluating the reason for equipment failure
- Evaluating and reducing costs of doing business
- Speaking about technical subjects to the company's clients or staff
- Providing technical assistance to attorneys working for clients involved in a lawsuit

Industry consultants are likely to find work from small companies that cannot afford to have someone full-time on staff to fill their intermittent needs, or they work for larger companies when specific expertise is temporarily needed in areas that those companies don't usually handle.

Resources
See also: Starting your own business; Writing; Computer-related jobs.
Groups
(Note: the address of many of these groups is that of the current Secretary or President; thus, these addresses may become outdated. Check the current *AVMA Directory* for current addresses).
1. Veterinary Consultants Network
Dr. Philip Seibert and Dr. Tom Catanzaro, Catanzaro & Associates, 18301 W Colfax, R-1, Golden CO 80401-4845, 303-277-9800

2. The Veterinary Hospital Managers Association
Provides a written and oral examination for certification in practice management; conducts an annual conference and other conferences throughout the US; provides job placement services. 48 Howard St, Albany NY 12207, 518-433-8911

3. Academy of Veterinary Consultants
Veterinarians involved in beef cattle medicine, herd health programs, and consultation. Provides continuing education (3 meetings per year, often in conjunction with larger veterinary conferences). Dr. Robert Sprowls, 6610 Amarillo Blvd West, Amarillo TX 79106, 806-353-7478; http://gpvec.unl.edu/public/avc/AVC.htm

4. American Veterinary Medical Law Association
300 N Clippert St Suite 4, Lansing MI 48912, 517-337-6401

5. National Speakers Association
Publications include *Professional Speaker* magazine. Offers training workshops and professional certification. 1500 S Priest Dr, Tempe AZ 85281; 602-968-2552; fax 602-968-0911; http://www.nsaspeaker.org

6. American Veterinary Health Information Management Association
Promotes the advancement of recordkeeping systems, information management, and personnel management via study, education and continuing education programs. Paula Wood, President, Oklahoma State University Veterinary Teaching Hospital, 1 BVMTH, Stillwater OK 74078-2041; 405-744-8574.

Courses/seminars

1. For specific information about *accredited colleges that offer distance learning*, and the subject areas taught, see the book list in Chapter 2.

2. The University of Illinois has a *multiple-weekend "Executive Veterinary Program"* that offers a *certificate in swine health management*. DVMs with two years of experience are eligible for the program. Twelve learning modules are offered every other month for three days each over a 2-year period. The training includes classes in consulting, leadership, economics, financial management, marketing, biostatistics, legal issues, nutrition, and epidemiology. *Executive Veterinary Program*, UI College of Veterinary Medicine, CEPS/Extension, 2938 VMBSB, Urbana IL 61801

3. The *National conference for agribusiness* is held each fall on the Purdue University Campus. Video cassettes and reports are available. 1145 Krannert Bldg., West Lafayette, IN 47907-1145, 317-494-4325, Fax: 317-494-4333; wall@agecon.purdue.edu

4. *The Agribusiness Seminar: a leadership workshop of the Harvard business school* is held in January each year. The Seminar is designed to help the experienced manager anticipate, and take advantage of, new trends and opportunities in domestic and international agribusiness. Focusing on long-range planning and coordination of the firm in its changing market structure, the seminar has as its central theme a concept of a world food system and the implications of global trends for private and public policy makers. Harvard Business School Executive Education office, 1-800-HBS-5577 (outside the US, dial 617-495-6555) Fax: 617-495-6999 executive_education@hbs.edu

Books

1. *The Consultant's Calling.* Geoffrey Bellman. Good reference; enlightening and fun reading. 1990.
2. *The Contract and Fee Setting Guide for Consultants & Professionals.* Howard L. Shenson. 1990.
3. *How to Develop and Promote Successful Seminars and Workshops.* Howard L Shenson, 1990.
4. *The Consultant's Kit: Establishing and Operating Your Successful Consulting Business.* Jeffrey Lant, 1996.
5. *Flawless Consulting: A guide to getting your expertise used.* Peter Block, 1981.
6. *How to Make at Least $100,000 Every Year as a Successful 7. Consultant in Your Own Field.* Jeffrey Lant, 1992.
Veterinary Practice Management. Dennis McCurnin, JP Lippincott, 1988.
8. *The Overnight Consultant.* Marsha Lewin, 1995. Contains good information despite the impossible title.

Periodicals

1. *Presentations* magazine focuses on how to give good presentations (speeches, seminars, etc—including the computer software to use to make slides). It's free for qualified subscribers (you must have some kind of influence in purchasing decisions). Lakewood Publications, 50 S Ninth St, Minneapolis MN 55402; www.presentations.com

Articles

1. *What it takes to become a consultant in your own field.* Profit Building Strategies for Business Owners, 20(7) 6/90.
2. *Shortcuts to starting a consulting business* (includes a list of information resources and an "aptitude test"). Sacha Choen. Training & Development 50(10) pp 38(7) 10/96.
3. *Selecting a consultant for profit and productivity.* Thomas E. Catanzaro. (Veterinary Practice Consultants, 303-277-9800).
4. *The veterinarian as an international consultant.* Stewart, D F Aust Vet J 48(5): 255-257, 5/72 (consulting for the UN-FAO, World Bank, etc)
5. *Consultant to the food animal industry.* Lawrence Price. JAVMA 190(10) 5/15/87 pp 1274-1276.
6. *The veterinarian: for emergencies only or consultant, too?* Rice, D. University of Nebraska, Nebraska Cooperative Extension Service, Lincoln, Neb. 1986 (86-220) pp 14-15. In series analytic: 1985-1986 Dairy Report.
7. *Evaluation of dairy heifer replacement-rearing programs.* (Consultant's role) Donovan, G. A.; Braun, R. K. Compendium on Continuing Education for the Practicing Veterinarian 9(4): p.F133-F139 1987
8. *The veterinarian's role as a consultant* (bovine practice). Morter, R. L. Modern Veterinary Practice 64(3): pp 226 1983
9. *Large-scale swine production.* Michael Terrill. JAVMA 198(4) 2/15/91 pp 563-565.
10. *Swine consultation practice:* A telephone and a computer modem. Gregg BeVier. JAVMA 190(2) 1/15/87 154-156.

CHAPTER 8

COMPUTER-RELATED JOBS

INFORMATION SERVICES / COMPUTER SOFTWARE

Working in information services or informatics is a combination of writing and computer work. Veterinarians can work with computers in several ways. Two basic categories are writing for database vendors and designing or writing content for software programs.

There are many services that provide indexes or abstracts of medical or veterinary literature. These services need people to review, index, or write abstracts of scientific literature, and to do literature searches. Other groups, universities, and companies have ongoing needs for literature searching, abstracting, or indexing. For instance, the National Agricultural Library has a policy of hiring people with science backgrounds as technical information specialists.

Companies that write computerized diagnostic programs may hire veterinarians to write some of the program content. Entrepreneur DVMs may also write their own software programs for sale to veterinary hospitals. Online vendors may hire DVMs to answer pet owners' questions or to write columns (*see* "Writing jobs").

These fields are rather new, so there's still room for people without formal training beyond the DVM to find informatics-type work if they have obtained the computer skills on their own. Also, many positions with the government combine these information skills with other work.

Information services

Veterinarians may be hired to help write abstracts or gather database information. Although library science professionals or technical writers are often used for this purpose, there is sometimes a need for a professional with the ability to understand medical terminology and complex studies. Veterinarians may be hired on a full-time or part-time basis, as employees or freelancers. Titles of full-time positions vary but include "research literature analyst" or "technical information specialist."

Daily work

Duties and basic qualifications include reading literature (sometimes in foreign languages); love of reading; basic computer skills (especially working with a database); and writing skills. This is a great job for people interested in learning about the latest information in their fields. The work involves a lot of reading and typing. Working indoors and at a desk could be a drawback for some.

Primate Information Center

An example of this type of job is one with The Primate Information Center (PIC), a bibliographic and reference service for researchers, laboratory animal, zoo, and exotic animal veterinarians. The PIC searches worldwide databases to obtain all published nonhuman primate literature, which is then indexed using the PIC's detailed thesaurus, into a computer database. The database holds over 90,000 records dating back to 1940. It is used for custom retrospective searches or monthly recurrent searches for individual researchers or veterinarians.

The Primate Supply Information Clearinghouse (PSIC), a PIC service, provides a communication network between research institutions, zoos, and biotechnology companies. The PSIC publishes a twice-monthly bulletin, *New Listings*, as well as providing a referral service.

Duties of the "research literature analyst" for the PIC include reading from a wide variety of journals, including those dealing with retroviruses and AIDS, then abstracting for a database all the veterinary and biomedical articles mentioning nonhuman primates (about 250 a month).

National Agricultural Library (NAL)

As one of the most comprehensive sources of US agricultural and life sciences information, the AGRICOLA (Agricultural Online Access) Database contains bibliographic records for documents acquired by the National Agricultural Library of the USDA. AGRICOLA serves as the document locator and bibliographic control system for the NAL collection, covering the field of agriculture in the broadest sense. The NAL hires Technical Information Specialists for indexing. Veterinarians would be desired as indexers for the veterinary literature.

NAL jobs are advertised through the USDA (these jobs are listed under "Technical information specialist," not "veterinarian"). Foreign language ability is not required, but computer skills and the ability to use online databases are necessary. The NAL is located in Maryland; indexers can work out of their homes part of the time but must come into the office a day or two a week. Pay varies with experience but ranges from GS 9 to 12. (*See* Federal Government section for pay scale explanation, and how to search for government job openings.)

Computer software

Veterinarians may work with computer software in two main ways: writing programs, or performing sales or technical assistance for a software company. Veterinary software includes diagnostic programs, business management programs, herd health monitoring programs (dairy production, nutritional analysis), and database programs (journals, abstracts, or seminars on disk).

Up through the 1990s, most veterinarians doing this type of work have been self-taught. As the area becomes more specialized and the amount of technical expertise becomes greater, it is likely that many DVMs doing this type of work will have had additional training in the area (by on-the-job training or by taking classes).

Daily work

Computer work is necessarily an indoor, desk job. The low level of contact with animals (and sometimes people) is desired by some DVMs; others manage to balance their love of computers with a need to interact with people, by working in sales or technical support. These jobs provide great mental stimulation and an easy way to keep up on the latest information in veterinary medicine. Pay depends on the type of company or government job held.

Internet job searching

"Veterinarians who are job hunting and who don't know how to use the Internet will miss a lot of opportunities. You can access employment listings from universities, biotechnology companies, and more through the Internet." —*Dr. Cathy Johnson-Delaney, Primate Supply Information Clearinghouse.*

To apply: information services or computer software

Look for jobs:

1. In the Federal Government (see "Federal jobs" section). Contact the Office of Personnel Management and look for jobs in "technical writing" or "information services." Potential hiring agencies might include the National Library of Medicine (NIH), the National Agricultural Library (USDA), or the National Technical Information Service (Dept of Commerce).

2. In the classified ads of newspapers of large cities.

3. Contact database companies (See the AVMA *Directory* for a list of names and addresses.)

4. Chat with industry reps at any large veterinary convention. Look for displays of companies that make diagnostic software or databases.

5. Attend meetings of the associations listed in this chapter's Resource list.

6. Start your own business. You could sell computer consulting services, a software product that you designed, or your services as a journal abstract writer.

7. Attend the Medical Library Association's annual meeting, and chat with database vendors in the exhibit hall (see MLA listing, below).

8. Attend the Special Library Association's annual meeting, where the National Technical Information Service meets (see listing, below).

Informatics Training and Courses

Informatics training is offered at many universities. Among them is the *health informatics training* offered at the *University of Missouri in Columbia* (573-882-6966), where short-term fellowships are available for veterinary students, and two- to three-year programs are offered for graduate DVMS. The Virginia-Maryland Regional College of Veterinary Medicine and the University of California at Davis also have informatics programs. The AVI (*see* Resources) keeps an updated list of similar courses in its newsletter.

The Stanford Section on Medical Informatics offers a one-week introductory course on Medical Informatics, held at the Stanford campus each summer. The course includes lectures, computer labs, and research project descriptions/demos. Each day is devoted to a specific topic in medical informatics. There are morning lectures and afternoon hands-on computer laboratory sessions and project presentations and demonstrations of medical informatics research at Stanford. (415)723-6979; short-course@smi.stanford.edu
http://www-smi.stanford.edu/shortcourse.html

Resources

See also: Federal jobs: CDC Public Health Informatics Fellowship; APHIS-VS (Animal health database, Center for Animal Disease Information and Analysis (CADIA), and the National Center for Animal Health Information Systems (NAHMS)); Writing jobs: writing for Web sites and online services; International jobs with the UN; Consulting jobs.

Groups

1. The Association for Veterinary Informatics (AVI) promotes the use of informatics by veterinarians; its newsletter includes information about informatics short courses and fellowships (for students as well as

graduate DVMs), as well as new software, computer resources, etc. Past
AVI newsletters may be found on the Web site. 1590 Augusta Ct, Dixon
CA 95620; 916-752-4408; fax 916-752-5680; jcase@cvdls.ucdavis.edu
http://netvet.wustl.edu/avi.htm

2. *The Medical Library Association* has a subsection for veterinary
librarians and a job placement service (free for members; a fee is
charged for nonmembers). Their annual meeting in May has educational
seminars (many focusing on computers and database searching) and
hands-on computer courses (you can buy tapes of the talks). The
meeting is worth attending for the exhibit hall alone, which is crammed
full of database vendors and suppliers. Go to the meeting to talk to them
about abstracting jobs; it's easier and faster than writing or calling each
one individually. MLA, Suite 300, Six North Michigan Ave, Chicago IL
60602-4805. 312-419-9094; fax 312-419-8950; info@mlahq.org
http://www.kumc.edu/MLA

3. The *International Conferences of Animal Health Information Specialists*
was originally organized by members of the Veterinary Medical Libraries
Section/Medical Library Association (VMLS/MLA) to enhance the flow of
animal health information worldwide. The conferences are directed to
librarians and other information professionals working in veterinary
medicine, laboratory animal science, and zoological and wildlife
medicine. Proceedings of past conferences are available. Sample talks
include:

• The role of information technology in providing animal health information—a publisher's point of view.

• A study of the animal health professional's use of information broker
services.

• Non-government information resource centers in the United States:
providing information on laboratory and field animal welfare.

• Databases and dynamic illustrations stored on microcomputer dis-
kettes as supplemental materials to books and printed media.
Contact Vicki Croft, Veterinary Medical/Pharmacy Library , PO Box
646512, Washington State University, Pullman, WA 99164-6512
(509)335-5544 Fax: (509)335-5158 croft@mail.wsu.edu or
croft@vetmed.wsu.edu

4. *The American Medical Informatics Association* is dedicated to the
development and application of medical informatics in the support of
patient care, teaching, research, and health care administration. They
hold an annual conference, a computer applications symposium, and
professional specialty group meetings; publish the journals, "Computers
and Biomedical Research," and "MD Computing," and offer discounts on
medical informatics software. AMIA, 4915 St Elmo Ave Suite 302,
Bethesda MD 20814; 301-657-1291; Fax 301-657-1296.
http://www.amia.org/

5. *Society of Technical Communicators* http://www.stc-va.org/
http://www.heron.tc.clarkson.edu/about_stc.html

6. *International Association of Business Communicators*
http://www.iabc.com/homepage.htm

7. *National Federation of Abstracting and Information Services* is an organization of the world's leading publishers of databases and information services in the sciences, engineering, social sciences, business, the arts, and the humanities, representing the for-profit, non-profit, and government sectors. NFAIS members are the international leaders in information collection, organization, and dissemination. 1518 Walnut Street, Suite 307, Philadelphia, PA 19102; 215 893-1561, Fax: 215 893-1564; nfais@hslc.org

8. The *Information Industry Association* represents companies involved in creating, distributing, and facilitating the use of information in print and digital formats. It represents the industry's interests in government policy and regulatory matters; promotes the industry and provides early awareness about new developments and emerging technologies; and provides a business development forum for interaction among top executives in the industry. The annual convention is a forum for interaction and debate on the most important business strategy and technology issues facing the information industry. It provides an opportunity to network with key executives from the world's leading information companies in virtually every segment of the information industry – publishers, database providers, online services, information distributors, systems integrators, Internet service providers, and a variety of other technology and telecommunications companies. There is a subsection for veterinary librarians. 1625 Massachusetts Avenue, N.W., Suite 700; Washington, D.C. 20036 (202) 986-0280; Fax (202) 638-4403   http://www.infoindustry.org/

9. The *Information Technology Association of America* (ITAA) is a trade association for those involved with information technology. It offers newsletters, meetings, and seminars. http://www.itaa.org

10. *The National Technical Information Service* is the official resource for government-sponsored US and worldwide scientific, technical, engineering, and business-related information. NTIS acquires information from more than 200 US government agencies including the USDA, EPA, and DHHS. Technology Administration, US Department of Commerce, Springfield, VA 22161; 703-487-4650

11. *The Society for the Internet in Medicine* promotes education of the public and the medical community in the applications of the Internet and related technologies in the fields of the medical sciences, healthcare practice and management. Members are eligible for reduced registration fees for Society events including MEDNET 97—The World Congress of the Internet in Medicine, and a reduction in the subscription to the journal "Medical Informatics." SIM Secretariat, School of Cognitive and Computing Sciences, University of Sussex, Falmer, Brighton, BN1 9QH, UK; +44 1273 678448; Fax +44 1273 671320 info-sim@mednet.org.uk http://www.mednet.org.uk/mednet.

Online

1. VETINFO is an Internet mailing list for discussing the topics of veterinary medical informatics and uses of computers in veterinary medicine. List Owners are Dr. Ken Boschert ken@wudcm.wustl.edu   and Dr. Jim Case jcase@gypsy.ucdavis.edu

To subscribe to the VETINFO mailing list, send e-mail to: listserv@wulist.wustl.edu

with the *body* of the mail consisting of the following (the command *must* be in the body, *not* the subject):

SUBcribe VETINFO Yourfirstname Yourlastname

2. Enter "technical information specialist" (include quotes) in Alta Vista or Yahoo (web search engines) to yield a list of job openings.

3. Vetlib-L is an online discussion list for veterinary librarians and those interested in the field. VETLIB-L@VTVM1.CC.VT.EDU

Books and Articles

1. Prescription for the Future: How the technology revolution is changing the pulse of health care. Andersen Consulting / G. Moore et al, 1996. Focuses on human health care, but has implications for veterinary medicine.

2. Career Options: Information Services. Article. Dr. Cathy Johnson-Delaney. (Research Literature Analyst, Regional Primate Research Center, Primate Supply Information Clearinghouse, Univ of WA, Seattle.) Association of Women Veterinarians Bulletin, 4/90.

CHAPTER 9

WRITING, EDITING, AND PUBLISHING

Although very few veterinarians make a living as full-time writers, writing is an integral part of any career path. For many DVMS, freelance writing is something they do "on the side" with their main income coming from other work.

Having your writing published can earn you the respect of your colleagues, spread the word about your other work, or give you a creative outlet. Whether you are writing full-time or "on the side," you must understand the business of writing.

FREELANCE WRITER

Magazine articles

Most veterinarians think of writing in terms of writing technical research articles for magazines such as JAVMA. In these cases, the writer is not paid to write; instead, the writer must publish in order to report research findings and to maintain his or her job in academia. In contrast, veterinarian freelance writers write for a living.

Veterinarians may write articles for a variety of magazines, journals, or newspapers. The full-time freelance writer is self-employed and has an office in the home.

Freelance writers begin by coming up with an article idea. The writer may call or write to magazines and ask for their "writer's guidelines," which outline the style and format in which articles must be submitted. The article's length, subject and style are considered when deciding which magazine to approach. A "query letter" is written to the magazine's editor, outlining the idea. The editor then writes or calls, and either turns down the idea or gives the assignment. If the article is assigned, the editor and writer discuss the payment terms and rights to be sold. A contract is then sent to be signed.

Veterinarian-writers usually write for two major markets: the veterinary professional journals, and magazines for animal owners. Veterinarians may write business or medical articles for a variety of professional journals, from *Veterinary Economics* to the *Journal of the American Veterinary Medical Association.* On a lighter note, they may write animal health care articles for magazines like *Bird Talk, Western Horseman,* or *Cat Fancy.* Although the latter articles may seem "simple" in subject matter, writing them is not as simple as it first appears.

Daily work

All freelance writers use a computer and word processing program. The work requires self discipline. The hardest thing about freelance writing is simply sitting down to write.

Writers often set a goal of sending out two or three query letters per week. They follow up on each if they haven't heard back in about four weeks. They set up a system that keeps track of all their ideas, letters sent out, and replies received, as well as assignments and their due dates.

Qualifications

To be successful, freelancers must be good at selling their work; being able to write is less important. The beginning freelance writer has two hurdles to overcome (besides being able to write well). The first is to actually send out a query letter or sample article. The next is to get over the rejection slips and editorial changes to your work. When it comes to editing, hold fast to being technically and medically correct, and be ready to give on stylistic editorial changes.

Veterinarian-writers don't have to be specialists to write well on a subject. Their DVM degrees *make* them "experts" in most people's eyes, when it comes to writing for pet or horse magazines. Also, whether their articles are directed at the lay public or veterinarians, they must use interviews with other experts to create a readable, credible, and interesting article. It's those interviews that create the illusion of the author as "expert." However, this means that non-veterinarian freelancers who do a good job of interviewing experts may compete with DVM writers for the same market.

Writing successfully requires studying the *business of writing*. This is different from, and just as important as, studying *how to write*. Serious freelance writers should take three steps: join a local writer's group; read the Writer's Market (book); and attend large writer's conferences (these are similar to large veterinary conferences, with seminars on the business of writing—from "What the magazines are buying" to "Understanding electronic rights").

Successful freelance writers have a good understanding of how magazines are published, what editors do, and what readers like to read. They study magazines so that they know the style, word count, and complexity of each magazine's articles. They then match each of their article ideas to the magazine where it fits best.

A brief overview of copyright for freelance writers

Freelance writers are self-employed writers who sell the *right to use* their work—articles or books—to magazines, book publishers, or veterinary-related companies. As a freelance writer, the first thing to know about your writing is that you own it until you agree otherwise, in writing. Copyright law stipulates that a work is copyrighted as soon as it is recorded in tangible form—whether printed or on computer disk.

Once you write something, you can sell partial or all rights to use your material. Most professional writers who write articles for magazines will sell only "first North American printed serial rights," which means the purchaser has the right to be the first one to use the material in printed form in a serial (magazine). Once they do so, you can then re-sell the material, at which time you are selling "reprint rights" or "second serial rights"—this means that the purchaser gets the right to use the material *one time*, but that it has already been used once elsewhere. Additional rights that can be sold include electronic, video, and foreign rights.

Doing "work for hire" means that you are selling all rights to your material to the person who hires you. People who write as part of their jobs as salaried employees are always doing work for hire. However, freelancers may also agree to do work for hire. Except for technical writing (see discussion below), this is a bad idea. Once you sell all rights to a work, someone else gets all the income from any future sales of that work. Magazines re-use your work in several ways. They can combine it with other articles on the same subject, and create a book; they can reprint the same article in several magazines; and they can sell the article online to computer users. If you sell all rights, you don't see a cent of the income generated for all those sales. A writer makes a living from the ideas generated in an article. The writer should, therefore, receive a part of any income generated by that material forevermore.

Many magazines attempt to get authors to sign a work for hire contract, agreeing only to something different if the author is smart enough to insist upon it. (It is *common* for writers to change the contracts they receive for writing an article or book. *Almost all contracts are negotiable.*) You should get extra money for every different form in which your work is published—including electronic forms. After all, the magazine is charging each reader for each of those forms, and you deserve part of that income.

Unless you write a piece that has no resale value, and is so specific and technical that you would never re-use it, don't sign a work for hire agreement. Or, if the magazine insists upon work for hire, you should insist on a fee that is considerably higher than what you'd get for the same article had you sold only first serial rights.

Many first-time writers worry that someone will "steal" their ideas for articles or books. Although this may occur, it is rare. The difficult thing to realize is that none of your ideas are original. Chances are that someone, somewhere, has thought of the same idea. So, when you send out a query letter, your goal is to convince the recipient that you are better qualified to write the piece than is anyone else, and that you have a unique perspective that will make the article fresh and original. If you've done a good job of that, there is no reason for the recipient to "steal" the idea and have someone else write about it.

Note: Veterinary specialists who work in academia, conduct research, and publish papers based on that research are not freelance writers. This work is always done as work for hire, for two reasons. First, the writing is done as part of their full-time jobs, as employees of the institution where they work (thus, even if the journal did not buy all rights, their employers would own the work). Second, most peer-reviewed, refereed journals that publish research studies have a policy of buying all rights to the material. This policy helps them ensure they are the first and only publication to "break the news," when or if that is important.

Pay

Writing articles does not pay well, partly because veterinary journals are accustomed to getting material for free—from academicians who must "publish or perish," or from veterinarians who don't know any better, and who sell their material for little or nothing. Pet magazines are similarly accustomed to getting huge volumes of material from pet-loving writers who are willing to write for low pay. As an example, most major pet magazines (e.g., *Cat Fancy; Horse Illustrated; AKC Purebred Dog Gazette; Western Horseman*) pay from $200 to $500 for an article (1996).

You cannot make a living writing magazine articles if you limit yourself to writing about pets or animals. Although you may be able to write an article in a day or two, you can't sell an article every day. The best you can hope for is that, at some point, you are hired to write a monthly column, so you get a regular but small trickle of income. (Once this happens, you are listed on the magazine's masthead as a "Consulting" or "Contributing" editor, a feather in your cap and something to put on your resume.)

There is more of a market for pet articles than just pet magazines. Many of the women's and "home" magazines also run articles about animals. The "Big" women's magazines (Good Housekeeping, Woman's Day, etc.) pay well for an article ($1000 and up). If you think you'll become a regular contributor, think again. There are thousands of freelance writers trying to break into these markets. There is no high-paying magazine that will look twice at your work until and unless you have published a *lot* of articles in smaller magazines, *and* you have become very well known (even for those silly basic articles about fleas or worms). Start by writing articles for your local paper and accumulate a few "clips" (samples of your work) that you can send to the pet magazines with your query letters.

The main reason to write is to help sell something else—another service you offer, or another product you sell. You can get a great deal of "free advertising" for your other products or services by writing articles on the same subject, and putting a plug in the author's bio (the short paragraph at the end of the article). For instance, the bio for an article in a cat magazine about litterbox problems could read: "Dr. Smith is the author of *101 Training Tips for Your Cat.*"

Another reason to write articles is to make a name for yourself. Perhaps you then want to augment your income as a speaker, a consultant, or in some other way.

Technical writing

Another outlet for freelance writing is technical writing for industry (pharmaceutical companies, pet food companies, etc.). In contrast to other types of freelance writing, technical writing is usually done as "work for hire." Also in contrast to freelance writing, it may be possible for veterinarians to make a living this way. Technical writers may be asked to sign a confidentiality agreement that stipulates they will not reveal company internal information for a specified number of years.

Some examples of technical writing include writing:
- The proceedings for a continuing education seminar
- A booklet or brochure about a product, for use by sales staff
- Promotional materials for a new product
- A publishable paper (for submission to a refereed veterinary journal), based upon raw data from a study

Daily work/pros and cons

The day-to-day work of a technical writer is similar to that of one who writes magazine articles: sitting at the computer in a home office, typing away. Instead of sending query letters outlining an article idea, you respond to a company that calls you and asks you to do a specific project. A computer, modem, and fax machine are essential in this business, as well as access to overnight delivery services such as Federal Express and UPS.

Technical writers rarely get public recognition for their work. They don't expect to see their byline above a refereed article they helped write, since the official authors of the study (the people who performed the study about which they are writing) will be the only ones listed (the writer may get a footnote of thanks).

Technical writers must have a good understanding of the goals of the company for which they write. If they are writing a piece for publication in a refereed journal, for example, they must be able to match the material with the most appropriate journal. They then write the article so it fits that journal's requirements. At other times they may be writing material for a sales booklet or brochure, which must be understood by its intended audience.

Writing allows you to interview lots of interesting people who are experts in their fields. You get to study and write about an incredible variety of fascinating subjects, some of which you'd never otherwise explore.

Pay

This type of work is far more lucrative than is writing magazine articles. It is customary to charge by the hour (from $25 to $100/hr, depending on your qualifications and the difficulty of the work), plus expenses (long distance telephone, computer research online charges, etc). It takes a long time to get established clients, so be ready for some lean years and keep another job on the side.

Read the section about copyright under "freelance writing." Copyright is less of a problem for technical writers than for magazine article writers. Most technical writing is done as work for hire, and this is not objectionable for several reasons. First, you may be writing confidential in-house materials for a company. Next, the material you write is so specific that there is virtually no reprint market for it. Also, most of the technical background information is provided to you by the company for which you are writing. And finally, the pay is high enough to justify the work for hire agreement.

To apply

Many large companies use their own employees to do their technical writing, but others hire outside freelancers for some or all jobs. One way to break in is to first call the company and ask if they do indeed hire freelancers, and if so, who decides when they are hired. Then write a letter directly to that person, including your resume and any clips of your work. Do not expect to be called immediately; however, your letter will be filed and you may be surprised with a call months or even a year or more later (especially if you've been contacting them a few times a year to ask if they have any work for you).

The best way to get work is by networking. Get to know people who work in industry by joining the *American Association of Industrial Veterinarians*, and following the other networking tips listed in the introduction and industry sections. There are also full-time government and industry jobs in technical writing.

Writing for Web sites, electronic mailing lists, or online servers

Writing content for online use is just another type of freelance writing. As part of a Web site or online provider's services, DVMs may answer questions posed by other online users (usually pet owners). It is important to define the number of questions that must be answered each week and the time frame in which questions must be answered. DVMS may also write regular columns, just as they would for a print magazine, or they may write informational articles that are indefinitely made available for pet owners searching for specific information online.

Almost all the information included in the sections about freelancing will apply to writing Web site content. Pay for writing used online tends to be low, and many contracts stipulate that the writing is done as work for hire.

For information about writing for computer abstracting or database services, *see* "Jobs with computers."

Writing a book

Many veterinarians have great book ideas in their heads. If you want to write a book, you must first answer this:

- Do you want to *make money* with this book (i.e., write something that sells)? Or,
- Do you just want to produce a book for the joy of writing and to get the information out to those who need it? Are you willing to *pay money* to do so?

The answers will totally change your approach to writing the book. If you are interested in writing a book that will sell, you need to study the business of book writing and selling. Start by reading the books listed at the end of this section, by joining your local writers' group, and by reading writers' magazines (see above discussion).

It is rare for a writer to start a career by writing a book. Few publishers will consider an idea presented by someone who has never published an article in a magazine. So, if you jumped to this section and skipped the section about writing magazine articles, go back and read that.

Many book authors have an agent. An agent represents the author, presenting the book proposal to a variety of publishers until it is sold. The agent then helps the author negotiate the book contract. Some agents continue to assist the author after a book is published, helping with marketing ideas and the selling of subsidiary rights (e.g., book excerpts sold to magazines, foreign rights). Use of an agent is optional, and depends on the amount of energy authors want to put into selling and marketing their books. Fiction books have a greater need for an agent's expertise than do nonfiction. (A publisher can more easily make a quick decision about a nonfiction book based on a book proposal alone, because the book subject and scope are readily apparent.)

Another option, self-publishing a book, should be undertaken only when the book's intended audience is small or occupies a narrow niche. Authors who self-publish a book because no publisher will buy it, often find that no one else will buy it, either. Successful self-publishing is done by experienced authors who have the time and knowledge to attend to all aspects of book production and marketing.

Because "writing a book" is rarely a career in itself, but part of the freelance writer's career, we won't go into book writing in detail. Once you enter the world of writing, attend writers' seminars, and read more about writing, the business of writing a book will become much more clear.

MAGAZINE OR JOURNAL EDITOR

There are a limited number of jobs available in editing veterinary publications. An editor is responsible for the content of the publication.

Daily work

Editing includes reading manuscripts that are submitted for publication; critiquing these and consulting with authors about changes and improvements (changes in style, sentence structure, scientific content, etc); deciding which articles to put in each issue, and how the issue should be organized; deciding about what types of columns or regular features to publish; reading letters to the editor, and deciding which of those to print; and doing some writing of your own, too. That translates to lots of time sorting through and reading mail; telephone time; writing lots of letters (to article authors, explaining rejections and revisions); and marking up articles as they are read, with questions, comments, and corrections for the author.

Editors spend most of their time at a desk, but their jobs are very much "people" jobs. Most editorial jobs require that the editorial staff lives in one place, where the magazine is produced (usually a city). A very few allow "telecommuting," including the position as editor of the AAHA Journal (*see* "Associations.")

Veterinarian-editors use their knowledge of veterinary medicine to decide what information is important enough to print, and thus to disseminate to other DVMS. In the process of editing, they are exposed to all kinds of interesting medical information.

Other kinds of editing: *Copyediting* is editing for grammar, punctuation, and spelling; this is usually delegated to a non-veterinary person. *Technical editing* is often delegated to specialists (e.g., submissions to JAVMA and AJVR are sent to specialists in the field—"reviewers"—for technical comments and suggestions for revision). Copyeditors and technical editors (reviewers) work with the magazine's editors, who have final say in whether or not an article is published. *Consulting editors, contributing editors,* and *editorial advisors* are usually freelancers, not staff (see "freelance writing," above).

Qualifications/pros and cons

Qualifications for editorial jobs include good writing skills, writing experience, love of words and reading, and an ability to interpret and analyze scientific studies for accuracy and logic. It is also essential that you are interested in working with people, and are able to give authors tactful, constructive criticism and advice in a positive and helpful manner. (Article authors sometimes have strong egos—especially when they are experts in their fields—and can be difficult to work with.) Editors should be comfortable with computer word processing and electronic mail. Editors of scientific and technical publications may need a background in research or knowledge of statistics.

The editor has to enjoy working with and supervising people, giving helpful corrections, and of course must love reading, writing, and words. The drawbacks include working with difficult authors, wasting time reading unusable material, and struggling to meet deadlines. Magazines that rely on advertising income have a delicate balancing act, in that there may be pressure not to print material that denigrates a big advertiser.

To apply

Job possibilities include *editor-in-chief, associate editor,* or *assistant editor.* The editor-in-chief of a magazine is generally someone who has worked as an assistant or associate editor at that or another, similar magazine. Your best initial approach may be to apply for a job as an assistant editor.

The Journal of the AVMA and the American Journal of Veterinary Research (both AVMA publications) have veterinarians on staff as editor-in-chief, associate editors, and assistant editors. All positions are located at AVMA Headquarters in Schaumburg, IL; openings are advertised in the Journal of the AVMA (but it's never a bad idea to get your resume on file, even if an opening is not advertised at the moment). The editor of the AAHA journal holds a part-time position and is not required to work at AAHA headquarters. (*See* Association jobs section.)

For information about potential openings with any other veterinary publication, write to the publisher or editor-in-chief listed on the magazine's masthead. Be sure to write to the address listed for editorial offices, and not the ones for subscriptions or advertising. Take a look at the mastheads of veterinary and pet journals to see which have veterinarians on staff.

PUBLISHING JOBS

Publishing and editing go hand-in-hand. Only a very few veterinarians work in publishing—that is, the business of getting a book, magazine, or journal typeset, printed, bound, promoted, distributed, and sold.

The publisher of a large magazine delegates work by hiring businesses that specialize in each area (e.g., printing, distribution, promotion). The publisher is the editor's boss, and works with the editor to make sure that there is content to fill each magazine. The publisher of a smaller magazine may be the editor-in-chief as well.

There are two basic ways to get into publishing. One is to begin a magazine or newsletter yourself. Another is to purchase a magazine from another publisher—that is, to buy the business. The work of publishing has little if any connection to veterinary medicine; even if you publish a veterinary work, you will spend the majority of your time managing the business, coordinating printers, advertisers, and writers, and managing your editors—not reading veterinary material. A strong background in editing and writing are necessary, as well as good business management skills.

MULTIMEDIA JOBS

Multimedia is a term that refers to the use of print materials, video, computers, and television to convey information. Many veterinary-related companies create their own multimedia materials (*see* "Jobs in Industry.") Others hire an outside firm to do this work. *Veterinary Learning Systems* is an example of a company that works to serve the multimedia needs of the veterinary profession. With four DVMs on staff, VLS is hired by a variety of companies to assist with marketing their products to veterinarians and their staffs. They create videotapes, books, CDS, scripts, and other materials. VLS also produces two journals, organizes meetings for companies, and assists companies with their customer service needs.

VLS' veterinarians are titled "Professional Service Managers," and their work includes a wide variety of tasks, from arranging space for meetings to editing technical material. Their jobs involve negotiating, working with people, and travel. They understand and are comfortable with marketing, enjoy writing and words, and spend much of their time on the telephone and answering mail. They constantly learn about new products and medications. More than half of their time is spent working at a desk.

GOVERNMENT POSITIONS

One sure way to make a good living as a full-time writer is to get a job with the government. You may be hired by any one of the main government agencies, from the Fish & Wildlife Service to the National Institutes of Health, as a technical writer. For more information, see the section on Federal Government jobs, or peruse the list of Federal job vacancies at the Office of Personnel Management's Web site: http://www.usajobs.opm.gov/

MEDIA WORK: TELEVISION AND RADIO

Media work is included here for completeness, not because it's a true career for veterinarians. Although veterinarians do appear on, or even host their own, television or radio programs, few are able to make this a full-time job with a focus on veterinary medicine.

Veterinarians who work with the news media do so for several reasons: to promote their other work (a book they're selling, or their veterinary hospital); for the fun of it; to improve their speaking skills; to improve their image to the public or their clients; or to help educate the public.

Because of the "aura" of television and radio, veterinarians who make such appearances are viewed by some of the public as special or exceptionally talented. After all, if they weren't special, why would the program be doing the interview? That statement is only partially true. The reality is that knowing the right people, making the right contacts, and being able to speak clearly, with animation, and in "sound bites" are important factors in getting on television or radio programs. For television, a good visual presence is important—professional-looking clothing, neat hair, and quiet body language (no fidgeting).

Let's say you are a consultant or a writer, and you want to make some news media appearances to help sell your book or consulting services. Or perhaps you are a housecall veterinarian, and think you can get lots of new clients by appearing on the local news. Because there are so many more radio than television stations, it will be easier for you to get on a radio show.

The first question to ask is this: What programs are your potential customers watching or listening to? Unless you have written a pet care book that is directed at the general public, there's no point in appearing on the *Today* show. Besides, they won't give you a second look unless your book is selling exceptionally well or is really different.

Start by either searching the Web or going to the library and looking up the names and addresses of local or specialty television and radio shows. (Specialty shows include television and radio segments devoted to pets or livestock.) Send them a press release announcing your news (you must have some news, or there's no reason to have you on). An example might be an announcement about your new housecall service and how you offer free classes on bird care at the local senior citizen's center. Another announcement might be that your new book, *101 Training Tips For Your Cat*, just received an award, and you and your trained cat will be hosting a book signing at the local bookstore.

Follow up your press release with a phone call. If you're scheduled for an appearance, ask about what you will be expected to discuss and how long the interview will last. You can even volunteer to send a list of "typical questions" that they might ask (this is normal, and makes their work easier). During the show, remember that it will be impossible for you to say everything you want to say, so don't try. Make sure the main receptionist has your contact information (listeners who want to contact you will call the station; the person who answers the phone should have your name, address, and phone number handy). Video- or tape-record all your appearances or radio interviews, and listen to them to learn from your mistakes.

Resources
See also: Jobs with computers—abstracting; Consulting.
Groups
1. All writers should join their *local writers' group*. Look for a group that focuses on the business of writing nonfiction. Watch your newspaper's community calendar for a listing of a writer's group. If you don't find one, ask at your library or call the newspaper. (Even if you join a national group, you should still join a local group).
2. Attend a *writer's seminar*. Note seminars listed in Writer's Digest magazine. Attend these just as you attend veterinary continuing education meetings. This is essential, don't skip it.
3. *American Society of Journalists and Authors*
A national organization of independent nonfiction writers who have met the Society's standards of professional achievement. 1501 Broadway #302 New York, NY 10036 (212)997-0947; Fax: (212)768-7414; 75227.1650@compuserve.com http://www.asja.org/

4. Council of Biology Editors, Inc. (CBE)
The Council of Biology Editors was established in 1957 by joint action of the National Science Foundation and the American Institute of Biological Sciences. It now functions autonomously with more than 1,200 members. Its purpose is to improve communication in the life sciences by educating authors, editors, and publishers; provide means of cooperation among persons interested in publishing in the life sciences; and promote effective communication practices in primary and secondary publishing in any form. Any individual interested in the purpose of the CBE is eligible for regular membership. 60 Revere Drive, Northbrook, IL 60062, 847-480-6349 Fax: 847-480-9282; cbehdqts@aol.com

5. American Medical Writer's Association
Produces a monthly "job market sheet" with lists of freelance, part-time, and full-time jobs for medical writers and editors. 9650 Rockville Pike Bethesda, MD 20814-3998; (301)493-0003

6. The Cat Writer's Association
Has many veterinarian members. Newsletter and annual meeting with educational seminars. Amy Shojai, CWA, PO Box 1904, Sherman TX 75091; 903-868-1022;
http://www.geocities.com/Heartland/Hills/5272/cwa.html

7. The Dog Writer's Association
Has many veterinarian members. Newsletter and annual meeting. Secretary Pat Santi, 173 Union Rd, Coatesville PA 19320
http://www.prodogs.com/dwaa/dw00001.htm

8. The Association of Industrial Veterinarians
(Join if you want to do technical writing, to get to know people in industry). PO Box 488, Oskaloosa, KS 66066-0488

9. American Agricultural Editors Association
Denise Clark, 612 W 22nd St, Austin TX 78705; 512-474-2041

10. Society for Technical Communication (STC)
The Society for Technical Communication exists "to engage in scientific, literary, and educational activities designed to advance the theory and practice of the arts and sciences of technical communication through the development of better educated personnel in the field of technical communication." Its 20,000 members include technical writers, editors, graphic designers, videographers, multimedia artists, and others whose work involves making technical information available to those who need it. STC, 901 N. Stuart St., Suite 904, Arlington, VA 22203-1854; 703-522-4114; FAX 703-522-2075, http://www.stc-va.org/

11. National Association of Agricultural Journalists
312 Valley View Dr, Huron OH 44839, 419-433-5412

12. Small Publishers Association of North America
PO Box 1306, Buena Vista CO 81211-1306, http://www.SPANnet.org

13. Publishers Marketing Association
Assistance for anyone who is self-publishing a book of any kind. Newsletter includes information about all aspects of book production. Cooperative mailings save lots of money. Annual "publishing university" is a 2-day series of seminars in editing, marketing, design, finance, law,

sales, and publicity. 627 Aviation Way, Manhattan Beach CA 90266; 310-372-2732; Fax 310-374-3342; PMAOnline@aol.com http://www.pma-online.org

14. *The Association of American Publishers*
Conducts a course in publishing scholarly journals, among others. 71 Fifth Ave, NY NY 10003; 212-255-0200; http://www.publishers.org

Online

1. *American Society of Journalists and Authors*
The ASJA Web site provides invaluable free information to freelance writers, such as contract tips, current facts and fiction about electronic publishing, and a chronology of ASJA *Contracts Watch,* which is an excellent source of news and information about publishers contracts and concessions on electronic rights. http://www.asja.org
ASJA's Contracts Watch is available by E-mail (dispatches only, no discussion). To join, send the following E-mail command:
To: ASJA-MANAGER@SILVERQUICK.COM   Message text: JOIN ASJACW-LIST

2. *Business forms and copyright information*
http://www.courttv.com/legalhelp/business/intellectual/copyrights.html
http://www.courttv.com/legalhelp/business/forms/940.html

3. *National Writers Union*
The NWU Web site provides analysis of electronic media and the future of copyright, and responds to concerns about access to information. http://www.igc.org/nwu/

Books

1. *Writer's Market* (Writer's Digest books. Get current year.) Contains names and addresses of book publishers and agents; how to write a query letter, all about copyright, how to target your market, and all the basics of the business of writing; and lists hundreds of magazines (their pay scale, the types of articles they accept, and the name and address of the editor to write to). Available in any large bookstore.

2. *ASJA Handbook: A Writer's Guide to Ethical and Economic Issues.* American Society of Journalists and Authors. ASJA, 1501 Broadway #302, NY NY 10036. (Discusses copyright, standard contracts and agreements for articles, books, and technical writing).

3. *The Editor-In-Chief: A practical management guide for magazine editors.* B. R. Patterson & C. E. P. Patterson. Iowa State Univ Press 1997.

4. *Business & Legal Forms for Authors and Self-publishers.* Tad Crawford. Allworth Press 1990.

5. *Complete Guide to Writing Nonfiction.* Edited by Glen Evans. The American Society of Journalists and Authors/Harper & Row publishers.

6. *Handbook of Magazine Publishing.* Folio, Stamford CT. Cowles Business Media.

7. *How to Write & Sell a Column.* Julie Raskin. Writer's Digest Books, 1987.

8. *How to Edit a Scientific Journal.* C.T.Bishop. ISI Press 1984.
9. *The Newswriter's Handbook: An introduction to journalism.* M.Stein & S Paterno. Iowa State Univ Press 1997.
10. *The Self-publishing Manual.* Dan Poynter. Para Publishing (has lots of other materials for self-publishers). PO Box 8206-222, Santa Barbara CA 93118-8206; 805-968-7277; Fax 805-968-1379. http://www.ParaPublishing.com
11. *Elements of Technical Writing.* Joseph Alvarez. Harcourt Brace Jovanovich 1980.
12. *How To Write A Book Proposal.* Michael Larsen. Essential reading. Do what it says, don't skip anything, and you'll be successful.
13. *How to Be Your Own Literary Agent: The business of getting your book published.* Richard Curtis. (This is must reading, whether or not you want to have or plan to have an agent). Houghton Mifflin 1984.
14. *Negotiating a Book Contract.* Mark Levine. Moyer Bell 1988.

Articles

1. *Practice or perish? My path from practice to marketing to editing.* Tim Phillips. JAVMA 202(8) 4/15/93 pp 1222-1224.
2. *Writing is no mystery to veterinarian.* K Baumgardner. DVM Newsmagazine 11/96 pp 30 (veterinarian who writes mystery novels).

Periodicals

1. *Writer's Digest.*
2. *The Writer.*
Pick up a copy of either magazine at your local magazine store or grocery. Serious writers should subscribe to one or both.
3. *Folio: the magazine for magazine management.*
4. *Publishing News.*
The above 2 are published by Cowles Business Media 203-358-9900.

CHAPTER 10

CAREERS IN VETERINARY "INDUSTRY" (COMPANIES THAT SERVE THE VETERINARY PROFESSION)

Veterinary students often hear the words "veterinary industry" and visualize a negative picture of a pet food sales representative. That unfortunate stereotype could not be more wrong. Let's start by getting rid of the word industry and being more specific about these jobs.

There is a wide variety of companies that make products or perform services for veterinarians and pet owners. These include medications; medical supplies; medical equipment; pet foods; laboratory supplies, equipment, and services; and insurance (for pets and livestock). Veterinarians are hired in every business that manufactures, provides, or distributes these products and services. These veterinarians may hold a DVM degree alone, or they may also hold additional degrees.

Approximately 1500 veterinarians are employed in veterinary industry. Because of corporate mergers and buyouts in recent years, the total number of jobs is shrinking. Pay is generally good, with excellent benefits.

A higher percentage of graduates from the following veterinary schools are employed by industry, compared with other schools: Iowa State; Kansas State; Michigan State; Ohio State; and the University of Pennsylvania. The Virginia-Maryland Regional College of Veterinary Medicine now has a Department of Corporate and Public Practice.

Daily work

Some of these jobs allow you to continue to work with animals, or pet and livestock owners; others allow you to interact with other veterinarians. All require that you use the knowledge you gained in veterinary school, even if it does not involve hands-on animal work. Job duties range from technical support (providing information about the company's products to veterinarians) to management (directing other DVMs or researchers in the company) to clinical research. Many of these jobs require extensive travel. Positions are available in several departments or areas.

Typical departments that employ veterinarians

Research and development
Quality control
Production
Product registration
Regulatory affairs
Marketing
Sales
Technical service

To get promotions and advance your career, you should, over time, take jobs in more than one of the above areas and should be willing to move between companies or to other parts of the country. Often, a higher salary or promotion means advancing into a management position, which takes you farther away from working with animals, animal owners, or veterinarians. Many veterinarians elect not to pursue promotion because they prefer to live in one place and are happy with their jobs.

Every company will have slightly different job descriptions, duties, and titles. One job in company A may have an entirely different title in company B and be divided into two jobs in company C. The descriptions that follow are included to give you a peek at the potential choices.

Pros and cons

Working for any veterinary-related company will invariably mean that you must already live in, or be able to move to, the city where your services are needed (that's not always the company's headquarters, though, especially for technical services jobs). The number of veterinarians employed by industry in 1995 was highest in New Jersey, Pennsylvania, Michigan, Kansas, and California. There are jobs with veterinary companies in every state, though.

No matter what your specific job, you represent the company for which you work—so you should have a positive opinion of their products, services, and business goals. Many jobs allow you to continue to work with animals and/or to have contact with practicing veterinarians. Pay and benefits are excellent, and there is plenty of opportunity for advancement (as with government jobs, the more you are willing to move, the faster you will advance). Many industry jobs involve a lot of travel.

All corporate employees are evaluated periodically by measurable performance criteria. For instance, you may be required to write a list of goals for each year, and your raises, bonuses, and promotions are based on whether you achieve your goals. Since there is always more than enough to do, you must learn to focus on the important tasks.

Pay

Veterinarians working in industry consistently earn higher salaries than do DVMs in any other category of work. Board-certified DVMs or those with additional degrees also see the most financial benefit from their training if they work for industry. The *American Association of Industrial Veterinarians'* annual survey for 1995 showed that the average salary for industrial veterinarians with a DVM degree was $84,886. Salaries tended to be higher in companies focusing on pharmaceuticals, health products, and poultry products, and lower in companies focusing on animal feeds. Salaries are higher for management positions. Most jobs in industry provide exceptional benefits, which add a significant sum to the total income.

Job Title	Mean Salary	% of Respondents
Director	$112,819	21%
Manager	$ 84,096	21%
Technical services	$ 72,000	23%
(Several miscellaneous categories made up the rest.)		

Primary nature of job	Mean Salary	% of Respondents
Management	$113,786	32%
Technical services	$ 77,813	29%
Sales/ marketing	$ 71,071	10%

Qualifications

All of these jobs require an ability to work within the structure of a business organization, including following all the company policies and procedures. You should enjoy working as part of a team, and be interested in keeping up your knowledge of company products and the associated diseases or management problems. Basic computer skills and good writing and speaking skills are necessary. Experience with a wide variety of animal species and a background in statistics are helpful. Knowing how to interact with the media is useful. Companies often send their employees to speaker training or media training workshops.

Some jobs require a few years of experience in practice, whereas others require sales, managerial or research experience. If a position looks good to you, but you lack the experience, take a lower-level job and gain the experience as you work. Good communication skills (telephone, interpersonal and group speaking, and writing) will increase the inexperienced person's chances of being hired.

One thing that veterinary industry is *not* looking for is a veterinarian who just wants to "get out of private practice." What company would hire someone because they want to get *away* from something else? Instead, they're looking for people who *want to get into the business*, i.e., those who have a positive reason for change. They want people who may still like private practice, but who are looking for a greater challenge.

To apply

Tip from an insider: *Jobs in industry are filled through a network. Who you know is important.* This needn't be a roadblock; just because you don't know anyone today doesn't mean you can't meet people. Go to any large veterinary meeting, and chat with the people working in the exhibit area (when they're not busy with Real Customers). How do they like their jobs? What other jobs are available in their company? Where do they live, and how much do they travel? Tell everyone you know that you are investigating jobs in industry.

If you currently have a job in private practice, chat with all the sales reps who come in, and ask them if they have a technical services DVM riding with them (who may be waiting in the car); then, talk to that DVM. Say *yes* to offers to go out to lunch. Offer to do clinical research in your hospital for the company.

Join the *American Association of Industrial Veterinarians* (see chapter resources). Attend their annual meetings, breakfasts, or luncheons at every veterinary meeting you can.

The person who has the most influence on hiring is *not* the person in the human resources or personnel department. (Note: I got no replies—that's zero—to letters I sent to large companies' human resources departments to gather information for this book. Once my approach changed to talking with specific people, I got the information I needed.)

Focus on companies you consider to be reputable and strong, carry good products, and whose DVM employees you would like as colleagues. Find out as much as you can about the company before you make your approach. Get their literature, brochures, and annual report. Look up their financial data in your library's reference department.

Peruse veterinary journals for advertisements. You can also find jobs through the AVMA Placement service (*see* Chapter 1). Follow up on your networking and your applications with a letter or E-mail. Call or write after you send out your resume, and call again every three to five months to remind them of your interest. Often headhunters call people in industry, looking for someone to fill a position. If you have been persistent, your name will be remembered and passed along.

Don't turn down a job just because it's not the exact one you want. Once you have "industry experience," your choices are much wider. Why not work for a year or two as a technical services rep, for example, if it gives you a leg up when you want to apply for a job in R & D?

Technical/professional service

Technical services is a good place for a veterinarian to start in a career in industry. From here, you can advance to other jobs .

A *Technical Service Representative* (TSR), *Regional Technical Manager* or *Professional Services Manager* learns the technical details about a company's products, and uses that knowledge to answer customer questions or to train sales people for the company. TSRs give seminars for sales staff and for practicing veterinarians, where they speak about their company's products or services (usually speaking in a broader sense of the disease, disorder, or injury that creates a need for that product or service; e.g., pet food company TSRs will give talks about nutrition in relation to health and disease). The TSR may "ride along" with sales representatives on their daily rounds to veterinary clinics, helping them answer questions and teaching them about the veterinarian-customer's concerns. They also represent the company to schools and colleges, and at veterinary meetings.

TSRs spend 50% or more of their time traveling; a company car is sometimes provided. Many give more than 50 lectures per year. The company may provide a set of slides and information to be given in a talk, but the TSRs often rearrange the material to suit their needs. TSRs must become experts in the medical or surgical area in which their company's products or services are used. They may be in charge of handling complaints about a product, including the follow up for each.

Qualifications include willingness to travel, and interest in, and preferably experience with, sales, marketing, and customer relations. (Veterinarians who have been in private practice usually have this experience.) The ability to write and speak well is a basic requirement, as is computer literacy (being comfortable using computers; extensive knowledge is not generally required).

Insider tips on getting a job in industry

• A method that is *not* likely to work when used by itself is to send a resume and cover letter to the personnel or human resources department of each company. Sending a letter to the technical services director may yield better results.
• Don't go to a headhunter firm yourself to look for a job; headhunters look for people who aren't desperate, but who are happily working somewhere. If you call them, you appear desperate. Networking is what makes you visible to the headhunter.
• The "kiss of death" is to say you hate your current job. If you hate practice, you will hate working in industry. Employers in industry want people who like practice but are looking for new challenges.
• Jobs in industry are filled through a network. Who you know is important.

Answering telephones (as a *telephone consultant*) can be a big part of technical services. Non-DVMs are assigned to telephone duty to screen calls, so that the DVMs handle only the calls that require their expertise. The DVM provides information to pet owners, veterinarians, journalists, breeders, and universities about the company's products or services, and may mail out printed information after a telephone conversation.

The telephone consultant may interact with company workers in R & D, marketing, or the packaging/labeling department to help answer caller's questions. In some companies, veterinarians may be assigned to do only phone duty (at least one pet food company hires veterinarians part-time on a contract basis for this purpose). Other companies have their regular TSR staff rotate through phone duty (e.g., one week on phone duty, then several weeks traveling).

A *Technical Affairs Manager* is responsible for a budget, strategic planning, and supervising other people. The job involves less travel than does the TSR position.

The *Director of Professional Services* is in charge of the Technical Services Department.

Research and development (R & D)

R & D is the area to explore if you still want hands-on work with animals and have an interest in clinical medicine. Many positions are open to DVMs, although some require additional training. Some R & D jobs allow you to stay in one place, but others require travel. Compared with some other industry jobs, the hours of some R & D jobs can be long since there are often deadlines to be met. Veterinarians with these jobs must be comfortable with the company's use of animals in research.

Basic research often requires specialists such as veterinary pathologists, toxicologists, and laboratory animal veterinarians. However, clinical research can be done by a DVM with clinical practice experience. The DVM in R & D should have a working knowledge of statistics and study design, obtained via an MS degree, research work during veterinary school, or even on-the-job training, by starting out as an assistant on another DVM's research project.

The R & D *Facility Veterinarian* manages the animal facility, including care and feeding of a large number of animals, treatment of sick or injured animals, and practicing preventive medicine (exams, vaccinations, etc). The Facility Veterinarian monitors the use of animals in research projects to be sure that experiments are both necessary and appropriate, and makes sure the facility passes inspection by meeting Federal requirements. In most cases this person has advanced training in laboratory animal medicine. (*See* Traditional practice—laboratory animal medicine specialty; FDA jobs.)

The *Biological Staff Veterinarian* is involved in project planning and monitoring, including deciding what animal species is best to use for a study; how many animals should be used; what special conditions should be provided; and deciding the best way to perform the experiment. Duties might include looking for adverse signs, drawing blood samples or performing necropsies.

A *Clinical Research Coordinator*'s job can include designing a study and then enrolling private practitioners, who then enroll their own patients. The work includes traveling to the practitioner's clinics to educate them about their role and to monitor the study; negotiating contracts with those practitioners; handling problems that arise during the study (side effects in patients); and then compiling and analyzing the data and generating a final report. The job can involve travel from 25-75% of the time. The rest of the time is spent on the telephone and at the computer.

The *Director of Research* manages a group of researchers dedicated to finding new products for animal health. An extensive research background may or may not be required, but knowledge of research is important. Training may be obtained on the job, and includes knowledge of statistics and how to set up a research study. Many companies will hire a DVM because of the practical, "real life" point of view this person brings to the research setting. The Director makes management decisions, writes budgets, and directs research (specialists do the actual research)—focusing on the business feasibility and common sense of each project. The Director tells the researcher what's needed, and the researcher tells the director how they can best achieve that goal.

Regulatory affairs and product development

The regulatory affairs department is in charge of all communication with the appropriate regulatory office (usually the FDA). The *Regulatory Affairs DVM* or *Product Development Manager* takes a new drug concept to the FDA and negotiates with that agency about the work that must be done to get it approved (including the types of studies—toxicity, field efficacy, or dose titrations; how many animals must be used; and duration of the study). That information is given to the clinical research department, which writes a study protocol that meets the FDA's requirements. The FDA then reviews these protocols, which are renegotiated to everyone's satisfaction before the study can begin. FDA approval also depends on developing package insert information and a label for the product. (*See* Government jobs, FDA)

Regulatory affairs jobs involve mostly desk work (writing, computer, telephone). These DVMs must keep up on developments in government regulations and in new products similar to the ones they are bringing to market. As with R & D, meeting strict deadlines may create long working hours. One must have the patience to deal with government regulations and government workers. Knowledge of laws, medicine, R & D, and the needs of practicing DVMs is important. One route to jobs in regulatory affairs is by working in R & D.

The *Product Development Manager*s oversee the entire process. They work with the formulations chemist to make the drug to the stringent regulations the government requires. In order for the product to meet specifications, the analytical group develops tests to analyze its content. The PD manager works with the toxicology group to determine safety for animals receiving the drug as well as for people handling the drug. Some companies have a team that may include a manager and field investigators. They may contract out a study to a university, with supervision by the field manager. The PD manager is not an entry-level position, but a *Field Product Coordinator* or *Field Monitor* could be. A variety of backgrounds would be appropriate for these positions, since the work differs with every project.

Sales and marketing

Sales jobs involve traveling to potential buyers (veterinary clinics) to present product information and to take orders. Additional marketing staff work to present a company's product to the veterinary profession as a whole (this work may include advertising and promotion). Although DVMs can fill these positions, most sales and marketing people are non-DVMs. These jobs are suited to people who are interested in organizational tasks, working with people, and traveling. They do not involve clinical medicine, but do require interacting with practicing veterinarians. Jobs in marketing require experience or additional education in that field.

Business development

Business development workers look for potential new products, make deals with other companies for cooperative ventures or buyouts, and perform other business services. Usually these people have business degrees, but a technical background is also necessary.

International positions

Companies with offices overseas may have openings for DVMs. Qualifications for these positions include experience in a multinational company; an understanding of the international differences in animal health markets, product development requirements, and scientific approaches; and exposure to colleagues in other countries. Foreign language is often not required.

How will you get the necessary experience? Get a job in the US working for a company that has offices in other countries, so you know their goals and methods of operation; or, take a temporary position with an international assistance group (*see* Chapter 12). Practicing veterinarians can host an international student through the International Veterinary Student Association; this may lead to an opportunity to visit that student's home and learn about the country (contact your area's veterinary school for information).

Sample job announcements

Scouring recent journals revealed a wide variety of advertisements for positions in industry. Here are excerpts of some of those, to give you a better idea of where you're headed. Remember that you can get the required experience by taking a lower-level job in the industry and working your way up.

> • *Manager of Regulatory Affairs, Animal Health*
> Pharmaceutical company. Involved in the preparation and
> execution of regulatory submissions, especially those dealing
> with claim extensions of existing products, including commu-

nicating with regulatory agencies to expedite the approval process, assisting preparation of regulatory strategies, and assisting in regulatory support for clinical development. Requires DVM; excellent oral and written communication skills; computer proficiency. Prefer 2 yr experience in regulatory affairs.

• *Companion Animal Technical Services Veterinarian*
Pharmaceutical company. Involves providing technical advice and information to DVMs and their clients, participating in new product development, and conducting clinical trials. Requires superior communication and interpersonal skills; DVM; 3 yr experience in clinical practice, industry or academia with expertise in small animal medicine. Up to 40% travel required.

• *Technical Service Veterinarian*
Pharmaceutical company. Provides technical support of all company products and support of R & D field activities. Requires 2 yr experience with swine and dairy cattle, and a working knowledge of companion animal medicine. About 60% of time is spent traveling. Oral, written, and human interaction skills necessary.

• *Research Veterinarian*
Pharmaceutical company. Involves the discovery and evaluation of animal health products for food and companion animals; conducting safety and efficacy studies in various animals, especially cattle and swine; working with infectious disease models; and providing veterinary services for animals at the research center. Requires DVM with experience in conducting experiments with large animals, knowledge of experimental design, statistics and regulations, and excellent communication skills.

• *Product Development Manager*
Pharmaceutical company. Involves coordination of several projects involving cattle, swine, and poultry products. Duties include designing efficacy and safety studies, coordinating efforts with product development and marketing departments, providing technical advice on assigned projects, and monitoring studies required in an animal drug submission. Postdoctoral experience and knowledge of US registration procedures is desirable.

• *Manager of Veterinary Services*
Pet food company. Summarize and interpret technical data, and provide technical information to the public and company personnel. Requires 3 yrs clinical experience, knowledge of research procedures and ability to understand marketing concepts.

• *Manager, Animal Development*
Pharmaceutical company. Manage several product development managers assigned to coordinate the R & D and Marketing efforts for new and existing animal products. Requires
strong managerial skills and experience in research and in
product development.
• *Animal Care Center veterinarian*
Pet food company. Provide veterinary care for research animals, including emergency treatment, surgical procedures,
vaccination, disease treatment, physical exams, and dentals.
Conduct clinical evaluations of animals during studies; visit
and monitors studies performed by outside research facilities;
give presentations on research studies, pet nutrition, and pet
food products; write summary reports of tests and evaluations
conducted; and assist in writing technical training material
and technical papers for publication. Requires 2 yrs of clinical
practice and 1-3 yrs of applied experience in animal research.
• *Professional Services Veterinarian*
Pharmaceutical company. Provide technical consulting and
guidance to practicing DVMs and to company's sales, marketing, R & D, and regulatory affairs groups; investigate and
resolve product related complaints; make technical presentations at veterinary and producer meetings; and represent the
company at industry seminars and veterinary schools. Requires 5-7 yrs of clinical experience in companion animal
practice or bovine feedlot practice. Prior experience in professional services, technical services or clinical research is
desired.

Resources
See also: Chapter 1(How to apply for any job); Government jobs (FDA).
Groups
1. AVMA *Membership Directory and Resource Manual*
Published annually; includes current and updated addresses of many of
the groups or associations listed throughout this book.
AVMA, 1931 N Meacham Rd, Suite 100, Schaumburg IL 60173-4360,
800-248-2862
2. *American Association of Industrial Veterinarians*
Dr. Steve Joseph, Secretary, Po Box 390, Shawnee, KS 66201, 913-268-
2554
3. *American Association of Pet Industry Veterinarians*
Dr. Dennis Cloud, 9418 St Charles Rock Rd, St Louis MO 63114, 314-
429-6666

Online resources

You can access a list of job openings of just about any company by visiting their Web site. To find Web sites, type in the company name using a search engine. Include the name in parentheses to limit your search to just those specific words in their specific order, e.g., "Novartis Animal Health" (Search engines are located on Web sites such as Yahoo and Alta Vista; consult a computer-savvy friend for help the first time you use one).

Books

VPB: Veterinary Pharmaceuticals & Biologicals. Veterinary Medicine Publishing Co, 9073 Lenexa Dr, Lenexa KS 66215. Includes names and addresses of companies that manufacture and sell veterinary medications, supplies, and pet foods.

Articles

1. *Industrial veterinary medicine: Career in a young company.* David Schabdach. JAVMA 197(12) 12/15/90
2. *Changes in the number and geographic distribution of US veterinarians employed by public or corporate organizations, 1980-1990 and 1990-1995.* Brad Gehrke. JAVMA 209(8) 10/15/96 pp 1404-1405.
3. *Veterinary clinical nutrition.* Rebecca Remillard. JAVMA 193(10) 11/15/88 pp 1238-1240.
4. *Industrial medicine in the land of Oz.* Elizabeth Hodgkins. JAVMA 195(7) 10/1/89 pp 922-923 (working for a pet food company)
5. *Present and potential perspectives for veterinarians in international careers (industry).* D. Mark Keister, Rhone Merieux. JVME Winter 1996 pp 45.
6. *Technical service careers: qualifications, responsibilities and opportunities.* Bruce Wren. Large Animal Veterinarian, Nov/Dec 1990 pp 27-30.
7. *Ready resource: Technical service veterinarians and you.* Bruce Wren. Pet Veterinarian Jan/Feb 1990 pp 20-22.

CHAPTER 11

ASSOCIATION AND ORGANIZATION JOBS

There are good opportunities for veterinarians to work in organized veterinary medicine. "Organized veterinary medicine" is a term used by veterinarians that refers to the associations that focus on veterinary issues. In addition to those groups with direct ties to veterinary medicine, many other livestock or animal-related groups may have jobs that a DVM could fill.

Associations that hire DVMs full-time include the American Veterinary Medical Association (AVMA), the American Animal Hospital Association (AAHA), and some state associations. Other potential employers include animal welfare organizations; state licensing boards (board members are usually volunteers, but the Director or Chair is often a paid position); the American Kennel Club (AKC); the Orthopedic Foundation for Animals (OFA certifies dogs of certain breeds to be free of signs of joint disease, and employs board-certified radiologists); the Delta Society (devoted to the human-animal bond); the National Cattleman's Beef Association; and the Morris Animal Foundation. *All these groups and more are listed in the AVMA Directory.* For information about jobs with international assistance organizations, see the next chapter.

These are primarily indoor jobs that include lots of telephone communication, reading, writing, supervising, and managing. Some positions require extensive travel and involve lots of meetings. Many allow for continual contact with veterinarians. Some positions that would be ideal for a DVM are not necessarily advertised that way, and many times the person responsible for hiring has a typical stereotypic view of "veterinarian," which may result in your being told that the group doesn't have any jobs for a DVM. Modify your approach to ask about any job openings at all, then see for yourself whether any are suitable for your talents.

ASSOCIATION DIRECTOR

The major *veterinary conferences* have become so large that their administration is a full-time job. For example, the Executive Director of the *Western Veterinary Conference* is a veterinarian. The *National Board Examining Committee for Veterinary Medicine's* Executive Director is also a veterinarian.

Although some *state veterinary associations* work with volunteer DVMs (hiring a secretary or office worker full- or part-time), others have a DVM on staff full-time, usually as the Director. Many state associations currently have a non-DVM as Director, but the position could easily be filled by a veterinarian.

Daily work

Day-to-day tasks include working on the computer, using the telephone, and conducting meetings. A lot of time is spent communicating with people (group members, journalists, members of related groups)—on the phone, by mail, by fax, by E-mail, or in person, at meetings. Travel is required (up to 50% of the time), both to conduct meetings for the association as well as to represent the association at various other meetings.

Pros and cons

Pros include working with motivated and outstanding members of the profession, working on a wide variety of tasks and issues, and keeping current on important issues facing the profession. There is no contact with animals, and there are stressful times as deadlines near and conflicts arise among constituents. Working hours are well-defined, although overtime and weekend work are occasionally necessary.

Organizational work dictates that you must always balance your personal opinion against the official position of the group, and you may have to work closely with people with whom you disagree on a particular issue. Meetings can become tedious, juggling many projects at once can be difficult, and the amount of time it takes to resolve issues can be frustrating.

Pay

The salary for these jobs varies widely. States with a low population may hire a part-time Director for as little as $15,000 per year; full-time positions could pay four times as much, or more. Benefits are usually excellent.

Qualifications

Qualifications include experience in some kind of practice, excellent verbal and written communication skills, and an ability to work with people on complex and often controversial issues. A Director must have staff management and administrative skills (usually gained by performing those tasks in private practice, and by reading materials from and attending talks by practice management experts). Leadership skills are essential. The Director generally lives in the city where the association or group has its headquarters. A Director of a state association should have a history of working within the association in volunteer positions; the Director of a Conference should have experience working on the Conference Board.

To learn more, talk to veterinarians who are on state association committees or on a conference's Board of Directors. Getting on a board or committee is a good way to gain experience; these are part-time, volunteer positions. Once you are involved with a particular association, you will have a better idea of how to advance to a paid position.

JOBS WITH ANIMAL WELFARE ORGANIZATIONS

Several national humane or animal welfare organizations employ veterinarians on staff, including the Humane Society of the United States, the Massachusetts SPCA, and the American Humane Society. Other smaller non-governmental humane or animal welfare organizations may employ veterinarians on staff. Both administrative and hands-on animal work are possible. Details about hands-on work are found in the Government jobs chapters.

See also: Jobs with the city, state, or county government: Animal shelter veterinarian. Jobs with the Federal government: USDA-APHIS Animal Care.

JOBS WITH THE AMERICAN ANIMAL HOSPITAL ASSOCIATION (AAHA)

AAHA is a group whose mission is to enhance the abilities of veterinarians to provide quality medical care to companion animals, and to maintain their facilities with high standards of excellence. Member veterinary hospitals are certified by the association if they meet stringent criteria for excellence.

The AAHA employed 5 DVMS as of 1997: the Executive Director; Management and Hospital Services Director; Hospital Services Manager; Practice Consultant; and Journal Editor. American Animal Hospital Association, 12575 West Bayaud Ave, PO Box 150899, Denver CO 80215-0899; 303-986-2800. http://www.acmepet.com/aaha/

The Executive Director

The Executive Director works out of the Denver office and is appointed by the Board of Directors. The current Director is a DVM who worked as a volunteer committee member with the association for many years. His duties include personnel management, financial management, and administration and management of all meetings, publications, and other member services and programs. The Director carries out the policies, programs and budget established by the elected Board of Directors. The Director attends AAHA board meetings and conferences.

Management / Hospital Services

The other two DVMs working out of the Denver office are in the Management Services / Hospital Services area. One is the organization's *Management and Hospital Services Director*. This person, who holds MBA and DVM degrees, provides management and financial and insurance services to members; conducts hospital surveys; directs the Practice Consultant team; and oversees the consulting program.

The *Hospital Services Manager* plans and directs the Hospital Survey Program; supervises and trains Practice Consultants in the completion of hospital evaluations; informs AAHA members of deviations from standards and assists them in compliance; and performs hospital surveys. She provides telephone and in-house support, responds to information requests, assists the membership division in recruitment, and speaks at meetings.

Practice Consultant

The *Practice Consultants* (only one of whom currently is a DVM) work in various areas of the country and are responsible for AAHA's on-site hospital evaluations. The Practice Consultant evaluates veterinary hospitals to assure adherence to the AAHA standards; acts as an ambassador of AAHA; and provides practice management assistance to members. He maintains an itinerary of hospitals to be visited, writes and files on-site reports, and promotes association membership. Computer literacy is required. Travel (flying and driving) are a major part of the job.

Journal Editor

The AAHA *Journal Editor* works part-time out of a home office; she is responsible for editing and producing the Journal of the AAHA. She solicits, reviews, edits and proofreads manuscripts; is responsible for meeting publication deadlines; directs manuscripts to reviewers; proofreads revised manuscripts and reviews journal layout; and attends committee and AAHA meetings. (*See* "writing jobs" for details).

JOBS WITH THE AMERICAN VETERINARY MEDICAL ASSOCIATION (AVMA)

The AVMA is the authorized voice for the veterinary profession. Its objective is to advance the science and art of veterinary medicine through programs of member service and public education. The AVMA runs on a lot of volunteer labor, but some paid positions are available in various AVMA Divisions.

The foundation of the AVMA is a series of *committees and councils* that are made up of volunteers (DVMs with other full-time other jobs, e.g., in private practice). AVMA council members are elected by a House of Delegates. Committees are established and appointed by an Executive Board. Committees and councils meet several times a year to work on specific issues.

The *House of Delegates* consists of volunteer representatives of 67 state and allied veterinary medical groups, each elected for a 4-year term. The House is approves the AVMA budget and decides on proposed amendments to the AVMA Constitution.

The *Executive Board* consists of DVMs elected for 6-year terms. These people are reimbursed for expenses, but their positions cannot be considered "jobs" in terms of making a living.

Committee and Council recommendations are sent to the Board for approval, and are then given to one of the AVMA *Divisions* for action. Here's where the DVMs employed by the AVMA take up the work.

Qualifications

Some positions within the AVMA require a specific advanced degree (e.g., MBA); others require only a DVM but also require specific experience and training (not necessarily a specific degree).

Most of these positions require some travel; all require working within a large organization, and communicating with a variety of other Divisions and outside groups every day. Most positions involve writing reports, attending meetings, and spending quite a bit of time on the telephone. Each Division must organize meetings of its assigned AVMA committees and councils, including preparing the agenda, setting up the time and place to meet (often on weekends), taking notes or minutes, preparing reports about the meeting, and then carrying out the directives of the committee or council as determined during the meeting. This could involve writing letters, setting up new meetings, arranging for speakers, or setting up a symposium.

Most of the Divisions are centered at AVMA headquarters in Schaumburg, IL. The Governmental Relations Division has its own office in Washington, DC. The following information was gathered from interviews and from reading actual job advertisements or announcements of jobs being filled, since official job descriptions were not available.

Pay and applications

Salaries are confidential and are not available. Benefits are good. Open positions are advertised in the Journal of the AVMA. You can also contact the Director of each Division, or the Human Resources Department at the AVMA, if you don't see an ad.

AVMA, 1931 N Meacham Rd, Schaumburg IL 60173; 1-800-248-2862; http://www.avma.org/   AVMA position announcements online: http://www.avma.org/membshp/jobs.html

AVMA Divisions and their employees

What follows is a brief description of each Division and its employees. *These descriptions are not all-inclusive, and they sometimes change.* For a current listing, look in the AVMA *Directory* under "AVMA official roster: Executive staff, headquarters."

Executive Division

Association Officers are elected each year by the House of Delegates (President-elect and VP) and Executive Board (Treasurer, Executive VP, Assistant Executive VP). The Executive VP and Assistant Executive VP are full-time employees of the Association. The President and President-elect receive a stipend, whereas the remaining officers are simply reimbursed for travel expenses. The Executive VP is the "CEO" of the AVMA; the President is the chief representative of the Association.

Scientific Activities Division

Positions held by DVMS include the *Director* and two *Assistant Directors*. *The Assistant Director* serves as the primary staff consultant to the AVMA Council on Biologic and Therapeutic Agents and its Drug Advisory Committee; implements AVMA policies and objectives related to the use and availability of drugs and biologics, and responds to member inquiries in that area; develops cooperative projects with national organizations; and maintains contact with government agencies, such as the FDA, FSIS, and USDA. (Background of current assistant director: previously employed as technical services DVM by a pharmaceutical company; associate DVM in a small animal practice; small animal internship.)

Publications Division

Positions held by DVMS include *Editor in Chief, Associate Editors* (several), and *Assistant Editors* (several), all with additional degrees. There is a trend toward requiring all editorial positions filled by DVMS with a PhD or board certification. Since most papers submitted to the journals are written by specialists, it is felt that the editors must have an equivalent depth of knowledge. *Assistant Editor* qualifications include research experience; and proficiency in scientific writing/editing and communicating. *See* "writing jobs" for details.

Membership and Field Services Division

Positions include *Director* and several *Assistant Directors*, one of whom is the *Head of the Career Development Center.* All of these are DVMS. This Division is responsible for getting the AVMA *Directory* updated and published every year; sending out dues notices, and collecting dues; maintaining the computerized membership list; and recruiting new members. The latter includes a lot of travel to veterinary schools to tell veterinary students about the AVMA, and to help the student AVMA chapters. The Career Development Center offers job matching and career counseling for AVMA members.

Education and Research Division

Positions held by DVMs include *Director* and *Assistant Director.* The *Assistant Director* implements AVMA policies and projects concerning education, research, animal welfare, euthanasia, specialty board certification and continuing education. He works with AVMA councils and committees, and calls upon communications skills for responding to questions and concerns from AVMA members and the public. This Division is also responsible for inspecting and reporting on veterinary colleges and veterinary technician schools, for their accreditation. Travel is required.

Governmental Relations Division (GRD)

Positions held by DVMs include *Director* and three *Assistant Directors* (formerly called Policy Analysts). The GRD staff monitor activities of the Congress and Federal regulatory agencies for issues of concern to the veterinary profession. They also provide liaison for the profession to the Federal Government and numerous Washington-based allied animal health and commodity group organizations. The GRD office manages the Congressional Fellowship Program (see below), and the AVMA's political action committee policy board (which decides which candidates will receive contributions from the AVMA).

The *Director* is responsible for the overall management of the GRD, including preparation of the Division budget. The *Assistant Directors* work with Federal agencies, congressional offices and veterinary and animal health organizations to address legislative and regulatory issues pertaining to veterinary biologics, pesticides, the safety of foods of animal origin, and animal drug issues. The current GRD staff veterinarians represent the disciplines of public health, food animal medicine, companion animal medicine, and biomedical research. Applications should be sent to the AVMA GRD office.

AVMA Governmental Relations Division, 1101 Vermont Ave NW, Suite 710, Washington DC 20005-3521; 202-789-0007; 1-800-321-1473.

AVMA *Congressional Fellowships*

The GRD also coordinates *1-year Congressional Fellowships* that are held by DVMs. Although this is a one-year position and not a long-term career, it can be an integral part of a career path in government or regulatory work. Fellows are not AVMA employees per se. This program is designed by the American Association for the Advancement of Science, and is sponsored by several scientific societies, including the AVMA. AAAS coordinates the program, sponsors a week of orientation activities for these individuals, and continues with dinner speakers throughout the year. Pay (1997) is $35,000/year.

Congressional Fellows serve as consultants, researchers, and scientific resources. They use both their pre-veterinary and veterinary expertise in advising others about scientific subjects. The job allows them to learn the details about US agricultural policy, and about agencies such as the Dept of Agriculture, the FDA, and others. Fellows attend an educational orientation program to learn about how the government branches work and the major issues facing the Congress that year. Then they are assisted in finding staff positions in the office of an elected member of Congress or with a committee. Duties might include holding meetings, writing letters, monitoring funding appropriations, drafting bills, and meeting with DVMs working for a variety of Federal agencies. This is a great way to get an overview of a wide variety of Federal jobs.

Potential jobs for former Congressional Fellows include working in any government agency; consulting with attorneys about policy and law in the area of agriculture or veterinary medicine; researching and writing policy analysis reports for private foundations or the government; implementing public education programs for food safety, risk assessment, biotechnology, and animal welfare; working for industry, in regulatory affairs; and lobbying (educating as a representative of groups, foundations, or industries).

Applications are due each December, and the fellowships start the following September. There are also 4-week student externships available; contact the same office for information.

Contact the AVMA GRD office for information.

Resources

Groups

1. American Society of Veterinary Medical Association Executives
Promotes cooperation and learning among administrative executives of
veterinary organizations; publishes a newsletter, a member profile book,
and a membership directory; hosts an annual public relations
workshop; and holds an annual continuing education session. Julie
Lawton, President; NY State VMS, 9 Highland Ave, Albany NY 12205-
5417; 518-437-0787; 74232.1707@compuserve.com
2. The American Society of Association Executives
Conducts "Association Management Career Seminars" where you can
learn more about a career in association management, and sponsors
continuing education meetings for association executives. It certifies
Association Executives who complete an examination and offer evidence
of successful association management skills. It publishes "Career Opps,"
a biweekly newsletter listing nonprofit openings nationwide in the
$30,000-50,000 compensation range (1997), and "Career Starters,"
listing openings compensating under $30,000 (here's a way to get a
"gain experience on the job job.") It has a resume critique service. 1575 I
St NW, Washington DC 20005-1168; 202-626-ASAE; fax 371-8825;
asae@asae.asaenet.org http://www.asaenet.org/
3. Meeting Professionals International
Professionals who plan or manage meetings for associations. 4455 LBJ
Freeway Suite 1200, Dallas TX 75244; 972-702-3000;
http://www.mpiweb.org

Articles

1. The world of association management. (Working for AAHA) John Albers.
JAVMA 191(8) 10/15/87 pp 944-945.
2. The Congressional Science Fellowship. Martha Gearhart. JAVMA 196(5)
3/1/90
*3. AVMA's Congressional Fellow enthusiastic over opportunities for
veterinarians in Washington.* Martha Gearhart. JAVMA 193:1496-1497.
4. Washington office staff addresses legislation affecting veterinarians.
JAVMA 203(10) 11/15/93 pp 1376-1380. (About the AVMA-GRD).
5. AVMA Washington Veterinary News is published by the AVMA
Governmental Relations Division. For a sample issue or subscription,
contact the AVMA GRD office.
   *6. An idea whose time has come: Veterinarians in humane society
administration.* Gary Patronek. JAVMA 202(6) 3/15/93 pp 862-864.

CHAPTER 12

INTERNATIONAL, VOLUNTEER, AND ASSISTANCE WORK

People who want to broaden their horizons, travel, or help others may find a niche in international, volunteer, or assistance work. These jobs include clinical veterinary medicine, public health, animal production and health, economics, and research. Most jobs are with government, service/assistance, educational, or religious organizations. There are likely to be openings in industry for DVMs with language skills and an interest in travel. For other international positions, also see the sections on industry, consulting, government, and military jobs.

A recent survey of international employment opportunities showed that about 75% of international jobs paid a salary, 15% relied on volunteer services but paid some expenses, and the rest paid no expenses at all. The survey also showed that about 20% of the positions required only a DVM degree, but the rest desired an additional degree (MS or PhD, often in public health or epidemiology). About half required fluent language skills, and 20% required minimal language skills (*See* Resources.)

Why work in a low- or zero-pay job? The skills and experience you gain may fill a void in your resume or give you that extra leg up on certain jobs. A short-term position may also provide you with a temporary break from your current job without taking the leap of leaving that job. You can use the time to reflect on your future goals.

For a wide variety of new opportunities, do a search of the World Wide Web, using the words *veterinarian* and *volunteer*. A recent search turned up interesting opportunities such as one in Cozumel (go diving, then work by helping out at the humane shelter there).

cozvac@cozumel.czm.com.mx; 011-82-987-24616, fax 011 -522-1774.

INTERNATIONAL PROGRAMS AT VETERINARY SCHOOLS

So far, these international programs are directed at students; however, opportunities for graduate DVMs may become available, including distance learning (via computer) and short courses. Through the efforts of Washington State University (WSU), a consortium among the colleges of veterinary medicine at Purdue, Texas A & M, Tufts, and WSU has been formed with the goal of enhancing foreign language and cultural abilities of veterinary students so they can effectively address global animal health issues. Each of the consortium members has established linkages with international institutions in veterinary medicine and the equivalent of the USDA in numerous countries. The vision is that veterinarians with knowledge in international animal health will provide needed expertise within state and Federal Governments, the corporate animal health industry, and as consultants to US livestock operations with international markets.

International externships for veterinary students are being established at universities, research stations, and pharmaceutical companies with offices in other countries. Classes offered at WSU to prepare students for these externships include "International veterinary medicine" and "Language and culture for international externships." For details, contact: Dean's office, WSU College of Veterinary Medicine, Pullman WA 99164; dean@vetmed.wsu.edu   http://vetmed.wsu.edu/

Other schools may provide similar opportunities. For instance, Tufts University has a program focusing on international veterinary medicine. The University of California at

Davis has an elective field course in comparative veterinary medicine that provides for an exchange of students between their school and one in Mexico. A student at the University of Illinois set up an externship with the Kiev Zoo, which included collecting donations of medical supplies in the US and taking them to the Ukraine.

Practicing veterinarians can host an international student through the International Veterinary Student Association; this may lead to an opportunity to visit that student's home country and learn about veterinary needs there. Contact the IVSA at your area's veterinary school.

A future goal of US veterinary colleges is to create a directory of resources for international contacts. To find out if this directory has become available, contact WSU (above) or:

Association of Veterinary Medical Colleges, 1101 Vermont Ave NW Suite 710, Washington DC 20005-3521.

INTERNATIONAL RELIEF (LOCUM TENENS) WORK

There is at least one international relief veterinarian list, called Vetlocums. This group uses the Internet to place announcements for "relief DVM wanted" or "relief position wanted." The Web site is arranged in categories: large/small animal practices, wildlife, exotics and international donor projects. They also list a calendar of international veterinary conferences; holidays for vets; and practices for sale. There is a small fee for placing an ad, but none to read the announcements.

Envirovet Ltd Ivy Wood, Westrop Green, Cold Ash, Thatcham, Berkshire RG18 9NW, England, UK +44-1635-202886; Fax +44-1635-202886; vetlocums@envirovet.demon.co.uk http://www.vetlocums.com/

Other international relief jobs are found on the variety of "job banks" online. As we've said elsewhere, Internet sites change continually. If you don't find these, search for more using the words "veterinarian" and "locum" or "relief."

1. Click on the "Europe" button at
http://www.showcom.com/user/vetjobs.htm
2. British free classified ads includes locum jobs in places like Hong Kong and Australia http://www.vetweb.co.uk/classads.htm

INTERNATIONAL CONSULTANT

After working for any of the organizations mentioned here, or in government jobs overseas, you may have the knowledge and the contacts to start your own consulting business. *See* "consulting" for details.

International consultant

"Getting parties to collaborate is a challenge, but it's a great opportunity to get people to put politics aside and to work together. Your political ability to articulate and persuade is what makes each project a success."—*Dr. Jody Garbe, International Consultant and former* USAID/AAAS *Fellow.*

JOBS RELATED TO THE ENVIRONMENT

This category of jobs didn't fit nicely into any particular chapter, but it falls under the category of "assistance" in a broad sense. Veterinarians who are interested in helping others through environmental awareness may find a niche in international work. Government jobs (with the EPA or FWS) might also be appropriate. USAID fellows also can have a positive impact on the environmental awareness of people in other countries.

A group called the *Alliance of Veterinarians for the Environment* (AVE) encourages veterinarians to get involved with careers that have a positive impact on the environment. The AVE is developing a career counseling project aimed at creating a "career changing tool kit" for DVMs wanting to find work related to conservation and environmental health. They will be including information on career paths that require further graduate training and their career focus targets environment related work.

Contact the AVE via Gwen Griffith, DVM, MS, Co-founder and President; 4801 Belmont Park Terrace, Nashville, TN 37215; 615-297-8925; Fax 615-297-8743; AVEGwen@aol.com or Leslie Dierauf, VMD Co-founder and Chair of the Board; 10 Sierra Lavanda, Santa Fe, NM 87501; 505-474-5810; Fax 505-474-5948; lesave@roadrunner.com or consult the AVMA *Directory* for a current address.

Also: The *Environmental Careers Organization*; Robin Boland, 29894 Windsor Court, Novi, MI 48377, 810-960-5857

AGENCIES AND ORGANIZATIONS WITH INTERNATIONAL POSITIONS

Heifer Project International (HPI)

Heifer Project International helps impoverished families worldwide become more self-reliant through the gift of livestock and training in their care. To help hungry families feed themselves, HPI provides more than 22 types of food- and income-producing animals, as well as intensive training in community development, animal husbandry, and ecologically sound, sustainable farming. Milk, eggs, wool, draft power and other benefits from the animals improve diets and supplement income, which pays for education, clothes, health care and better housing. HPI requires recipients to "pass on the gift" of one or more of their animals' offspring to other needy families. This practice builds self-esteem by encouraging recipients to become donors and multiplies the benefits of the original gift.

HPI has two veterinarians on staff in the US in paid positions: One is the Asia/South Pacific *Director and staff veterinarian*; the other is the *"WiLD coordinator"* (Women in Livestock Development). The latter position does not require a DVM. Both those jobs are located at the HPI headquarters in Little Rock, AR. HPI tries to hire local nationals in other countries, so that veterinarians are hired to work in their own countries. However, some opportunites exist for others to fill paid positions overseas.

The current Director has a background in international issues, including membership in a student international group while in school. His job includes extensive international travel, often in rustic conditions; dealing with animal health issues in tropical regions; public speaking and communicating by E-mail, mail and phone; and lots of paperwork. Experience with computers, cross-cultural situations, and development is vital for this type of work. Language skills and intercultural skills are extremely helpful. International travel is routine and can become a chore since the busy schedule and dealing with jet lag can be exhausting.

In addition to the paid positions, there are *volunteer opportunities* with HPI. You can participate in HPI's mission by volunteering at one of their three Learning and Livestock centers, one of the five regional offices, or the World Headquarters in Little Rock, AR. You might have the opportunity to visit an HPI project in another country as a participant in a work-study or study tour.

Volunteers in International Veterinary Assistance (VIVA) provides animal health care for Heifer Project International supplied animals, and for other livestock as well. Volunteer DVMS are occasionally needed.

Pros and cons / To apply

This is exciting work that includes helping people who truly need it, around the world. However, most jobs are not paid, and for those that are, the salary never gets very high—although benefits are usually good.

HPI/VIVA, PO Box 808, Little Rock AR 72203; 501-376-6836; 1-800-422-1311. http://www.intellinet.com/Heifer/Heifer.html or www.charity.org/heifer.html

VetAid

VetAid is a Great Britain-based international assistance group. Sample job announcement: "Animal Health Advisor, Gaza & Inhambane Provinces, Mozambique. VetAid requires a tropical veterinarian with relevant technical experience gained in overseas livestock development projects, to join our project team as Animal Health Advisor. The job will include developing the animal health components of the project including quarantining of imported cattle, disease surveillance using participative techniques, and rehabilitation of infrastructure. The contract is for 30 months with salary in the region of £15,000 - 18,000, taxed locally, plus pension, contribution to housing and health, and accident insurance benefits. Applicants should hold an appropriate veterinary qualification, have a practical approach and be available to start at short notice."

VetAid, Centre for Tropical Veterinary Medicine, Easter Bush, Roslin, Midlothian EH25 9RG, UK. Tel/Fax +44 (0)131 445 3129 or vetaiduk@gn.apc.org

The Peace Corps

Founded in 1961 by President John F. Kennedy, the Peace Corps is a US Government agency which places Americans in foreign countries that have requested Peace Corps volunteers. The three goals of the Peace Corps are to promote world peace and friendship; to help promote a better understanding of the American people on the part of the peoples served; and to promote a better understanding of other people on the part of the American people. Peace Corps volunteers work in a variety of fields, including agriculture, community development, education, business, health, nutrition, and natural resources. They fight hunger, disease, illiteracy, poverty and lack of opportunity around the world. The length of service, including the initial three months of training, is usually around 27 months, and the Peace Corps covers all living, travel, and medical expenses during that time.

While the need has remained for volunteers to work in agriculture, education, forestry, health, engineering, and skilled trades, countries are increasingly requesting help in new areas: business, the environment, urban planning, youth development, and teaching English for commerce and technology. Emerging democracies such as those of the former Soviet republics have turned to the Peace Corps for assistance for the first time, while previous Peace Corps hosts such as Chile and Ethiopia have reestablished relationships to address more advanced development issues.

*United Nations Volunteers (*unvs*)*

The unv program, which operates through the Peace Corps, was established in 1971 by the un General Assembly and is administered by the un Development Program. The US sends about 25 citizens per year to serve as unvs. Approximately 57% of un volunteers serve in Africa, 23% work in Asia and the Pacific, 12% work in the Middle East and the former Soviet Union and about 8% work in Latin and South America. Apply through the Peace Corps.

To apply

To be eligible for Peace Corps service, you must be an American citizen. There is no upper age limit. Married couples may serve in the Peace Corps, but both people must apply and be accepted and it is usually more difficult for the Peace Corps to place them. Those with dependent children are not placed. Most assignments require a Bachelors degree, some require a Masters, and some require 3-5 years of work experience instead of, or in addition to, a BA/BS. It is recommended that you apply at least six to eight months before the time you are available to depart in order to increase your chances of acceptance.

Applicants must fill out a medical history and undergo physical and dental exams since a health condition easily managed at home can become a serious medical problem in countries that the Peace Corps serves. Host countries do not often have US levels of medical care; sites can be remote, and assignments often are physically and emotionally challenging.

Peace Corps, 1555 Wilson Boulevard, Suite 701, Arlington, VA 22209-2405, (800) 424-8580; http://www.peacecorps.gov/

Christian Veterinary Mission (cvm)

The cvm works to "share the love of Jesus while practicing veterinary medicine" in countries worldwide. Veterinarians can help the cvm with long- or short-term missions. Short-term missions last 2-3 months and are self-funded. On assignment, you will perform basic livestock health, such as vaccination and deworming. Long-term missions are for three years, with two-year renewal options; projects focus on training local men and women to be village animal health workers. The current Director of cvm is a veterinarian.

cvm, Dr. Kit Flowers, Director; 19303 Fremont Ave North, Seattle WA 98133; 206-546-7201 rkf@crista.wa.com

Volunteers in Overseas Cooperative Assistance (voca)

voca is committed to enhancing the development and economic opportunities of cooperatives and agriculturally based enterprises. Most assignments suitable for dvms are related to large animals, especially livestock. voca assigns veterinarians for 2-12 weeks in volunteer positions worldwide. Dairy farm management projects could be filled by dvms with dairy experience; a recently filled position was for a cattle nutrition specialist; and a previous program used DVM volunteers to design veterinary programs for Albanian university students interested in ruminants, monogastrics and poultry. VOCA has been using quite a few veterinarians in recent years.

VOCA, 50 F St NW Suite 1075, Washington DC 20001, 202-383-496; West coast: 1-800-556-1620; VOCA-CALIFORNIA@voca.org Central: 1-800-386-2286; VOCA-WISCONSIN@voca.org East: 1-800-335-8622; VOCA-OHIO@voca.org

Rotary Club International

Rotary was founded on the basis of exchanging information with people in diversified careers, fellowship and community service. It quickly spread into international service. Rotary's Group Study Exchanges are small groups of young professional and business people in their twenties (typically four plus an older Rotarian leader). A 4- to 6-week exchange is arranged with a similar group from another part of the world, with an intensive program of visits involving many talks and presentations. Candidates for these visits are recruited by the district that sponsors them through the local clubs.

From a Rotary member: "Some of our scholarship recipients study veterinary science abroad, and some of the professionals who participate in our exchanges are vets. There have been some grants to developing countries to provide or improve care of livestock. However, most of our volunteers are in the human health care field (doctors, dentists, etc). who focus on medical care to people." Contact:

Your local Rotary group, or visit their Web site: http://www.rotary.org/

People to People Citizen Ambassador Program

People to People was founded by Dwight D. Eisenhower in 1956 and was originally administered by the US State Department. This private, nonprofit organization is dedicated to improving global understanding through international cultural exchange. It develops, organizes, and administers educational travel programs. The program arranges for adult professionals who have common interests to have the opportunity to travel abroad together with the purpose of meeting and exchanging ideas with international colleagues who have similar backgrounds, interests, and professions. Over the past four decades, the company has organized programs for more than 33,000 adult professionals.

Teams of scientists, agricultural producers, crop researchers, agricultural engineers, food processors and packagers, and veterinarians meet with their counterparts, lecture, perform on-site tests and evaluations, discuss recent technical advancements, and assist farmers, breeders, technicians, and researchers in less-developed, traditionally agrarian societies. Delegations also share the latest techniques with their counterparts in developed nations. These exchanges have led to significant research modifications, new technologic applications, and ongoing scientific, technical, and business collaborations. Participants must pay their own expenses.

Citizen Ambassador Program, S. 110 Ferrall St, Dwight D. Eisenhower Building, Spokane, WA 99202-4800 (509) 534-6200 Fax (509) 534-5245; api@ambassadors.com http://www.ambasssadors.com

The United Nations

Many organizations exist under the UN umbrella, and some of these offer job opportunities for veterinarians. See the UN Web site for details about the organization. Specialized agencies of the UN (e.g., FAO, UNDP, WHO) should be contacted directly for job information. To be considered for mid-level and higher posts, candidates must possess an advanced university degree (i.e., beyond BS), in addition to relevant professional experience. Normally, a minimum of six years of professional experience is required. Information on currently vacant positions is available on the UN Web site, as well as at UN Headquarters, UN Information Centers throughout the world, other offices of the UN family, the Foreign Ministry of the respective Member States, and certain educational and/or professional institutions (universities, women's associations, etc.). The Secretariat maintains a computerized roster of qualified candidates for these posts.

Also see: Peace Corps-UN Volunteers

UN Staffing Support Section, Division for Planning, Recruitment and Operational Services, Office of Human Resources Management, Room S-2555, New York, NY 10017 http://www.unsystem.org/

Employment info http://www.un.org/Depts/OHRM/brochure.htm

Food and Agriculture Organization (Web site has job postings)
http://www.fao.org

Animal Health Service, FAO
http://www.fao.org/waicent/FaoInfo/Agricult/AGA/AGAH/Default.htm

UN Headquarters internship program

The UN Headquarters Internship Program is offered to students enrolled in graduate school, with a view to promoting a better understanding of major problems confronting the world and giving them an insight into how the United Nations attempts to find solutions to these problems. The program consists of three two-month periods throughout the year. As the UN has no provision in its budget to pay interns, all costs connected with internships must be borne by the students concerned or by their sponsoring institutions or governments.

UN Internship Program Room S-2580, Division for Staff Development and Performance, Policy and Specialist Services, Office of Human Resources Management, New York, NY 10017.

FAO Agricultural Scientist

Job announcement: Animal Production and Health Section, Vienna. Requires DVM, PhD, or equivalent in animal production or veterinary medicine; 6 yr practical experience in animal nutrition/reproduction; working knowledge of radioimmunoassay and/or enzyme-linked immunosorbent assay; working experience in developing countries; fluency in English, French, Russian or Spanish; ability to communicate fluently in written and spoken English. Duties: Coordinate Research Programs in the field of animal nutrition/ reproduction, dealing with feed supplementation strategies, improvement of artificial insemination services, analysis of purine derivatives, and development of assays for tannin determination in leguminous plants; provide technical support for technical cooperation projects in the field of animal nutrition and reproduction; organize training courses; maintain a program for the use of RIA kits for measurement of progesterone; assist in the development and supervision of the technical aspects of the animal production and health program.

Dairy and meat officer

FAO, UN: Animal Production Service job announcement. Requires university degree and postgraduate specialization in animal production, agriculture, meat or dairy science (Note: DVM would probably qualify here.) Experience in training, extension or research or programs to enhance producer participation in development activities in developing countries. Working knowledge of English, French or Spanish, and limited knowledge of one of the other two. Ability to plan, organize and evaluate work programs, to write clearly and concisely, and to establish and maintain effective working relationships with people of different national and cultural backgrounds. Computer literacy and ability to use word processing equipment. Responsible for activities related to institutional development training in the dairy and meat sector, in particular to promote development of livestock product supply systems; plan and develop programs to ensure production of milk and meat of consistent quality at point of primary sale and promote appropriate pricing policies; adapt and transfer appropriate technology in meat and dairy development to member countries; organize and conduct scientific and technical meetings; prepare and edit reports. Salary US $60,984 to 82,600.

UN Peacekeeping Operations

This agency seeks professionals with proven track records, an advanced university degree or its equivalent in a relevant discipline, four years of relevant professional experience and fluency in English and/or French. Fluency in additional languages, such as Arabic, Portuguese, Russian or Spanish, as well as working experience in developing countries, constitute a definite advantage. Applicants must be in excellent health and prepared to work in hardship areas under difficult and sometimes dangerous conditions. They must also be available at short notice. Most missions are classified as "non-family" duty stations. The compensation package includes salary and an appropriate mission subsistence allow-ance, which has been established to cover living expenses while at the duty station. The UN Office of Human Resources Management maintains a computerized roster on which candidatures are kept active for assignments to Peace-keep-ing Operations. Interested applicants may obtain an applica-tion form from, or submit their CV to:

UN Personnel Management and Support Service, Field Administration and Logistics Division, Department of Peace-Keeping Operations, S-2280, New York, NY 10017.

World Health Organization and Pan American Health Organization

WHO and PAHO are continually seeking the services of highly qualified health professionals. The professional technical staff act as advisers in public health to Member Governments and, consequently, candidates must possess substantial training and experience in this field before they can be considered for an assignment.

The PAHO was established in 1902; in 1948, PAHO was fran-chised by the WHO as its regional office for the Americas. It serves as the specialized agency in health for the Organiza-tion of the American States and the United Nations. Within PAHO, the Veterinary Public Health program is under the Divi-sion of Disease Prevention and Control. This is a large, unique program with a staff of more than 200 distributed world-wide as follows: 5% at the headquarters in Washington DC; 21% inter-country and country advisors assigned to the different country offices; 65% at the Pan American Foot and Mouth Disease Center in Rio de Janeiro, Brazil; and 9% at the Pan-American Institute for Food Protection and Zoonoses in Buenos Aires, Argentina. Most of the staff are DVMs with post-graduate degrees in preventive medicine and public health.

Qualifications / To apply

Requirements vary depending on the position, but normally an advanced degree in public health is highly valued. In ad-dition, most adviser positions require at least seven years of experience at the national level and at least two years of par-ticipation in technical cooperation programs and activities, preferably in the American Region for posts stationed in the Americas. PAHO positions normally require fluency in English and Spanish. Knowledge of Portuguese and French is desirable. Language requirements are specified in each vacancy.

Sample job announcements, WHO

* *Resident Project Coordinator*, India. WHO Global tuberculosis program, Short-term Professional Vacancies. Coordinator of GTB's operational research project in India focusing on improving the quality of care in the private sector and responding to the research needs of a modernizing national TB control program. Requires three to five years public health experience in developing countries, plus primary health care or private health services management experience. Monthly Remuneration US $6,300.

* *Scientist*, Special Program for research and training in tropical disease, Geneva, Switzerland. Duties include providing overall coordination of all R&D in the filariases (i.e. onchocerciasis and lymphatic filariasis); ensuring that its drug discovery research component maintains an appropriate level of and vigorous activity in the filariases; managing Product Development Teams in the onchocerciasis and lymphatic filariasis area; developing plans, preparing budgets and reporting progress. Requires Doctoral degree in medical or biological sciences. Good publication record and success in fund-raising for research would be an asset. Knowledge of pharmaceutical R&D and particular experience in managing product development, including good practices. Broad knowledge of infectious diseases, including tropical diseases. Sensitivity to needs of disease-endemic countries and disease-control programs. Knowledge of onchocerciasis and/or lymphatic filariasis is an asset.

WHO Job vacancy page (Important: Look at vacancies titled "scientist." Also see the UN site for more vacancies.):
http://www.who.ch/programmes/per/vacancies/vacancy.htm
Pan American Health Organization (PAHO)
WHO Regional Office in the Americas (AMRO), 525 Twenty-third Street, N.W., Washington D.C. 20037; (202) 861-3396 or (202)861-3200; Fax: (202) 861-3379 or 202 223 5971; http://www.paho.org/
postmaster@paho.org
World Health Organization (WHO)
20, Avenue Appia, CH-1211 Geneva 27, Switzerland, Tel: (41-22) 791-2111, Fax: (41-22)791-2300 or (41-22) 791 0746; postmaster@who.ch
http://www.who.ch/ http://www.who.ch/Welcome.html
http://www.who.ch/AboutWHO.html

Other overseas opportunities

A wide variety of *service and church groups* may provide opportunities for short-term international work. Contact those in your area for more information.

Write to *veterinary schools in countries of interest,* and ask if there are any courses, internship or volunteer opportunities. For instance, the University of Pretoria in South Africa offers an opportunity for training in tropical diseases and parasites prevalent in Africa. Short courses (one week to one month long) vary each year; subjects might include veterinary laboratory diagnostics, African epizootic diseases, or wildlife immobilization.
Shirley Schroder (Course convener), Dept of Veterinary Tropical Diseases, Univ. of Pretoria, South Africa; shirley@op1.up.ac.za

The *Organization of American States Student Intern Program* is designed for junior, senior, and graduate students at the university level to allow them to work within their fields of study. The Program, although non remunerative, is highly competitive. In order to be selected, students must have at least a 3.0 GPA and a good command of two of the four official languages of the Organization (English, Spanish, French and Portuguese; preferrence will be given to the first two official languages).
OAS/Public Information, 17th St. and Constitution Ave. N.W., Washington, D.C. 20006; (202)458-3754; fax (202)458-6421
http://www.oas.org

You can get information about many groups through *InterAction, a coalition of over 150 US-based non-profits* working to promote human dignity and development in 165 countries around the world. In the US, these groups are called "private and voluntary organizations," or PVOS. InterAction coordinates and promotes these activities and helps to ensure that goals are met in an ethical and cost-efficient manner.

http://www.interaction.org/index.html or, for a list of the Web sites of all 150 groups, go to http://www.interaction.org/members.html

When approaching any of these groups, you may be turned away when you ask about positions for veterinarians (once again, the person you're asking may think of veterinarians as dog doctors). Instead, start by asking about positions related to agriculture or livestock management.

Resources

See also: Federal Government: USAID Fellowships.; Federal jobs (APHIS Veterinary Services, USAID, EPA, FWS); Military jobs; Industry; Consulting jobs.

Books

1. A *Directory of Resources for International Contacts* is not yet available, but its creation is a future goal of the Association of American Veterinary Medical Colleges. It will include a list of organizations or societies interested in veterinary medicine. Contact the Dean's office of your area's veterinary college to find out if this has become available, or the Association of Veterinary Medical Colleges, 1101 Vermont Ave NW Suite 710, Washington DC 20005-3521.

2. *Culture Shock! Working Holidays Abroad—a practical guide.* Mark Hempshell, 1996. Focuses on non-professional jobs, but includes good tips (listed by country) about work permits, entry visas, money exchange, cost of living, health risks, and cultural norms.

Articles

1. *The Internationalization of veterinary education: strengths, challenges, and opportunities.* Journal of Veterinary Medical Education (entire issue) Vol 23 Winter 1996. Special issue: Proceedings of the 14th symposium on Veterinary Medical Education.

2. *Employment in international veterinary medicine: A survey of requirements and opportunities.* M. T. Correa et al. JVME 22(1) pp 25-29, Spring 1995.

3. *Realistic international career opportunities for US and Canadian veterinary graduates.* D.M. Sherman, et al. JVME Winter 1996 pp 21-30.

4. *Enhancing international veterinary education through curriculum development.* JAVMA 209(7) 10/1/96

5. *A veterinary volunteer in the south pacific.* JAVMA 208(8) 4/15/96 pp 1216-1217.

6. *The Internationalization of veterinary education.* Primo Arambulo. JVME Winter 1996 pp 34-35. Discusses the Veterinary Public Health Program of PAHO/WHO.

7. *Present and potential perspectives for veterinarians in international careers (industry).* D. Mark Keister, Rhone Merieux. JVME Winter 1996 pp 45.

8. *Seven habits of highly effective globalized veterinarians.* Lonnie J. King. JVME Winter 1996 pp 48-50.

9. *The world's food supply and the role of food animal veterinarians.* JAVMA 210(6) 3/15/97 pp 751-752.

10. *The veterinarian's role in the welfare of wildlife.* James R. Scott, DVM. JAVMA 198 (8) 4/15/91 pp 1380-1385.

11. *The veterinarian as an international consultant.* Stewart, D F Aust Vet J 48 (5): 255-257, 5/72 (Consulting for the UN Food & Agriculture Organization, the World Bank, and others)

CHAPTER 13

TEACHING

Veterinarians know a great deal about a variety of scientific subjects. If you enjoy teaching others, you can get a job anywhere from a community college to a veterinary technician school.

COLLEGE TEACHING OR ADVISING POSITIONS

Veterinary specialists are employed by veterinary teaching hospitals to teach veterinary students. (*See* "Traditional practice" for a list of specialties.) However, only a portion of these jobs involves teaching. Universities usually require that their faculty members also participate in research projects, publish articles, and participate in committees and university organizations. Specialists must be board-certified and are encouraged to pursue a PhD or MS if they work in academia. Those who focus only on teaching are unlikely to receive tenure.

There are many other teaching jobs that can be filled by a DVM without additional training, and that don't require research work. Veterinarians may be qualified to teach a number of science, anatomy or animal production courses. They also may be hired as advisors for pre-veterinary or veterinary students.

Daily work

The advisor's work includes advising students about classes, obtaining the required veterinary experience, and writing vet school applications; conducting mock interviews; and supervising off-campus internships.

Teaching includes preparing course outlines, materials, and tests; assisting students during and outside class time; giving lectures; and keeping up on the subject taught. A teacher, as part of the faculty, is often required to participate in various committees and give occasional speeches to various interest groups.

Pros and cons

It's often rewarding to work with students who are interested in, and enthusiastic about, science or veterinary medicine. As a faculty member, you make great contacts within the university system; get perks like free E-mail; and are paid to expand your knowledge. Cons for those who are "only DVMs" include job uncertainty, the political environment in the university, and feeling a bit overshadowed as a DVM in a PhD world (the unspoken laws of success in the university are "PhD and publish"). Many jobs are part-time, which may include no benefits. There is little opportunity for advancement without an additional degree.

**Veterinary Career Advisor,
College of Veterinary Medicine.**

Job announcement. Faculty position at rank of lecturer; 2-year renewable appointment. Requires DVM; preference given to those with related experience/qualifications. Duties: advising students of career opportunities and curriculum alternatives, managing the job placement program, and acting as student liaison.

To apply

Some openings are advertised in JAVMA; others in the *Chronicle of Higher Education* (*see* Resources). Contact veterinary schools and ask about advisory positions.

WORKING WITH A VETERINARY TECHNOLOGY PROGRAM

Both part-time and full-time positions are available for DVMS as teachers in veterinary technician schools.

Director

The Director of a veterinary technician program is in charge of hiring instructors, coordinating the educational program, developing curriculum, proposing and managing a budget, and recruiting, interviewing, and counseling students. The Director often has teaching duties as well (lectures, laboratories, correcting papers, etc), but spends less time at this than do the teachers. Office work, meetings, and telephone time (talking to prospective students and to veterinarians trying to hire a technician) are part of the daily work.

Pros and Cons

The Director has conflicting roles: representing the needs and interests of the program to the administration, and representing the administration's policies and procedures to the faculty and students. Some Directors may feel that they have a lot of responsibility and limited authority. Pay is moderate but there are good benefits. The job is challenging and full of opportunities to explore new interests and to meet interesting people. Hours are regular and travel isn't usually required.

Educator/teacher

Veterinary technician educators teach a variety of medical and surgical skills to technicians. Many veterinary technician programs utilize community veterinarians part-time for lectures or for "laboratory" sites where students can get hands-on experience. However, all programs have at least one full-time DVM on staff. Teaching time includes lectures, labs, creating and grading class materials, and computer work.

Pros and cons

Veterinary technician educators have less hands-on animal contact than do private practitioners, but there is still a significant amount of teaching that involves working with animals (anesthesia, nursing care, and radiology labs). Salaries are often lower than those of DVMs in industry and government. Rewards include helping students learn and develop; a good benefits package, with scheduled vacation days; no emergency calls; and being able to teach subjects that you learned in veterinary school. Teachers and especially directors have to put up with the bureaucracy and red tape that come with any school or administrative job.

Qualifications / To apply

A background in mixed practice is helpful, since work with all species is taught. Directors need skills in administration, management, and communication. To find job openings, contact the Association of Veterinary Technician Educators, and write to the Veterinary Technician Schools that are listed in the AVMA *Directory*.

Resources

See also: Federal civilian and military jobs (with any agency, you can become a teacher of the skills you learn on the job, teaching other people new to the agency); Government jobs with the extension service (extension agents' jobs are as educators).

Job announcements

1. *The Chronicle of Higher Education* is a weekly tabloid that includes meetings, seminars, workshops, and classified employment advertising for teachers, higher education administrators, and faculty members. PO Box 1955, Marion OH 43306-4055. http://www.chronicle.com

2. Veterinary technician teacher openings are also advertised through the AVMA Career Development Center's *Job Placement Service*. Contact the AVMA for more information.

3. For a list of *Veterinary Technology programs at US schools* (there are 64 as of 1996), see the current AVMA directory. Write to each for information about job openings. Although there is more than one school in some states, 13 states have no veterinary technology program at all

(as of 1996)—including Alaska, Hawaii, Idaho, Montana, Arizona, and New Mexico.

Groups

Association of Veterinary Technician Educators
The 3-day AVTE Symposium is held every two years in the summer at different sites. It provides the opportunity to bring together veterinary technician educators from all over the North American continent. Subjects of talks include information for program directors (recruitment, finances), educators (teaching tips, distance education), and other pertinent issues. Attendance runs between 100-150 individuals. This is a good place to go to network (i.e., make contacts for potential future jobs, and find out what the work is really like).
AVTE President, Dr. Sharah McLaughlin; St Lawrence College, Veterinary Technology; Kingston Ontario K7L 3X8 Canada; 613-544-5400
(or see the current AVMA Directory, or the AVMA Web site, for current address)
The AVTE produces a *quarterly newsletter* that includes job announcements and information about new veterinary technician programs at various colleges.
AVTE Newsletter, Dr. Pete Bill, Editor; Veterinary Technology Program, Lynn Hall, Purdue University, West Lafayette, IN 47907

Articles

Directing a veterinary technician program. Karen Hrapkiewicz. JAVMA 190(12) 6/15/87 pp 1538-1539.

CHAPTER 14

GOVERNMENT JOBS

What do the words "working for the Government" mean to you? To me, they always brought up the image of a military veterinarian (who spent all his time inspecting meat), or a state veterinarian (who spent all his time reading health certificates). No wonder I never wanted to work for the Government!

The reality of Government work is far more varied than my stereotypic perception. Before you dismiss this option, read through the following sections carefully. There is a wide variety of jobs available that pay well, offer mental stimulation, and can still fill your needs for working with animals, if you so desire. Government jobs are some of the most underappreciated of all careers open to veterinarians. *The vast majority of the Government veterinarians interviewed were excited about what they were doing and loved their jobs.*

The titles or "official descriptions" of most Government jobs don't tell you a thing. (What does "in charge of disease control" mean?) No wonder most veterinarians don't have a positive view of Government jobs! Take another look, though: these jobs include small animal, equine, and food animal work; hands-on animal work; laboratory and research work; or management and supervisory positions.

General information about all Government jobs is discussed first, followed by specific agencies and the jobs within them. The exact job descriptions may change over time, but the general ideas remain the same. You'll need to be patient in reading these chapters, since understanding specific job descriptions requires a discussion of each agency's organizational structure. If you can wade through that, then you've passed one criterion necessary for Government jobs.

When considering Government jobs, remember to look beyond jobs that require a DVM, to those that simply ask for someone with a science background, or someone with a Bachelors degree that you hold (microbiology, biology, chemistry?). Think of your overall qualifications, not your degrees (you write well; have held supervisory positions; etc).

Pros and cons

Benefits of any Government job include good pay and great benefits, guaranteed raises, fairly regular hours, and a clear job description (i.e., you know what you're supposed to be doing). Field jobs allow you to continue to work with livestock and with ranchers and farmers, without many practice headaches (the type of animals you'll work with depends on the state, e.g., pigs in Iowa, cattle in Montana). Jobs can be located in rural or urban areas. Sometimes you can travel to interesting places. Once you get over the paperwork and bureaucracy, you can focus on the interesting parts of your job—whether that be pathology (food inspection), disease management, animal care, or herd health.

All Government jobs include lots of paperwork, policies, and procedures. Government veterinarians need to care about regulations (which most do, since they understand the reasons behind the rules). They must be able to write well, and be ready to fill out lots of reports. Travel is often required. Several Government workers have described their jobs as requiring a delicate balance between doing a good job, and *not* doing a thorough job. If they are too strict with regulations, they raise a fuss—and thus get complaints from the people or groups they are regulating, giving supervisors a headache. Another complaint is that they have to spend a certain amount of time *justifying* their own jobs, rather than *doing* them—to make sure that their positions are not eliminated.

The Government and many associations are very concerned about the "official descriptions" of various jobs. *Any job descriptions or titles listed here may be changed, so consult each agency for up-to-date information.* However, the descriptions here should give you a good idea of the types of work involved.

CHAPTER 15

WORKING FOR THE CITY, STATE, OR COUNTY GOVERNMENT

Approximately 700 veterinarians work for state or local governments. The greatest number are employed in Wisconsin, North Carolina, Florida, Texas, and California. A higher percentage of graduates of the University of California, Colorado State, Cornell, Iowa State, Michigan State, Ohio State, and Texas A & M work for state or local governments than do graduates of other veterinary schools.

CITY OR COUNTY JOBS

Many cities throughout the US hire veterinarians for positions in public health, animal shelters, or animal care facility inspection. The vast majority of the jobs are with animal shelters. Most animal care facility inspection is done by veterinarians with the Federal Government, but some facilities are governed by city regulations and thus undergo inspection by city veterinarians. (See USDA-APHIS-Animal Care for a complete description of the duties of an animal care facility inspector.)

City or county public health veterinarian

Cities and counties have Public Health Departments that may hire veterinarians. Contact your city or county Public Health Department for information about specific positions and their titles.

Sample job announcement: Public Health DVM

Public Health DVM for the County Department of Public Health, Environmental Health Division, Technical Support Section. Salary $23.28 to $26.11/hr (1997). Enforce laws relating to meat, poultry, and aquatic foods for the County area; provide professional assistance and advice regarding veterinary medicine to departmental units; formulate and interpret policy for the Meat Inspection Program; coordinate a rabies control and prevention program with the Communicable Disease Control Officer and Laboratory; and advise the medical profession on matters relating to rabies and other animal diseases communicable to man. Requires DVM with 2 years of experience, preferably in a public health agency or in public health inspection work. Should have a thorough knowledge of infectious diseases common to man and animals and of control measures for such diseases; knowledge of laws relating to animal control and communicable disease control; and knowledge of and skill in performing ante and post mortem examinations. An MPH is desirable.

Animal shelter veterinarian

Many animal shelters hire a full-time staff veterinarian. Some shelters do not hire DVMs at all, whereas others retain a DVM only on a part-time or consulting basis. Still others contract with a veterinary hospital to perform necessary procedures such as spay and neuter surgery.

The shelter DVM performs basic medical and surgical procedures on shelter animals; vaccinates animals; spays and neuters animals; identifies animals with tattoo or microchip; and euthanizes animals. Long-term or complex care is usually not performed, since resources must be concentrated on animals most likely to be adopted. Life-saving medical care, but not extensive care, is given to injured animals. Shelter DVMs are often called upon during disaster situations, and must be ready to handle large numbers of animals if necessary. They are often in charge of investigating claims of animal abuse. Shelter DVMs must be especially knowledgeable about animal behavior problems, disease transmission, kennel management, and vaccination protocols in high-risk situations. Shelter DVMs may be partially or fully responsible for staff management, budget preparation, fund raising, making public presentations (e.g., speaking to school children and other groups about pet ownership), and serving as a liaison with related groups (e.g., working with the local veterinary medical association to decide what medical and surgical care should be performed by the shelter vs. private DVMs).

Agencies that provide animal shelter can be public (supported by tax dollars); private (nonprofit, tax exempt, charitable agencies); or private agencies with a public contract.

Pros and cons

Laws regulate the specific actions of DVMs working for public agencies; these laws may sometimes conflict with what the DVM believes to be proper medicine. A board of directors is the "boss" for DVMs working for private shelters. The DVM working for a private agency with a public contract is directed by the law *and* a board of directors.

The shelter veterinarian performs a needed public service and promotes responsible pet ownership. Parts of the job can be intellectually challenging, including kennel management and working within a political structure. Cons include repetitive surgical work, performing a lot of euthanasias, constraints of a limited budget, inability to treat and follow through on complex cases, and a generally "bad reputation" among other practicing DVMs, who may see a shelter DVM as a threat to their livelihood (because of discounted services—spays, neuters, and vaccinations—performed at some shelters). Hours are fairly regular, although the shelter DVM may have to take emergency calls during evenings and weekends.

The *National Animal Control Association* published a list of "Pros and cons of working in the field of animal control" in one of their newsletters. Pros included the ability to protect pets and people; the joy seeing animals adopted by loving, responsible people; the gratification of assuring that impounded animals are being provided shelter and care; the peace of knowing that unwanted animals are at least provided a humane and dignified death; the excitement of unusual animal calls; and the friendships developed with other shelter workers all over the country. Cons included frustrations with irresponsible pet owners; lack of understanding by the public of the need for animal control and of the problems of animal overpopulation; stress from abuse by people and depression because of animal euthanasia; exposure to communicable disease and injuries by animals and humans; and sometimes long hours or being on call.

Pay
Pay varies by geographic area, but is generally as good as that of the average veterinarian employed in private practice. However, the benefits are excellent. For example, one large city pays its veterinarians $20-30/hour, plus full medical and dental benefits, retirement plan, tax-deferred child care, professional memberships, insurance, license fees, and more.

Qualifications / To apply
Most positions require only a DVM degree, but others may require management, public speaking, organizational, administrative or fund-raising skills, and knowledge of animal behavior and kennel management.

To add to your expertise, find out whether your local community college offers classes in human relations, city management, municipal law, or public relations. Read the literature about animal behavior. Join Toastmasters if you have trouble speaking.

Every city that has an Animal Control Department should have a DVM working part-time, full-time, or on a contractual basis. Call your local department to find out their situation. You may also see job ads in the publications of the groups listed below, local newspapers, the city's Web page, and veterinary journals. (*See* Association jobs:animal welfare groups.)

Animal care facility inspection (city, county, or state)

This is a job that includes inspecting facilities where animals are raised or cared for, such as dog breeding kennels, veterinary clinics, and research facilities with laboratory animals. Some cities take charge of inspections in their area; in other areas, DVMS hired by the Federal Government fill a similar role. State law or city ordinance defines which facilities are to be inspected, and by whom. In some states and cities, there is no provision for inspection of veterinary hospitals. In some cities, a shelter DVM is also responsible for animal facility inspection. *See* the Federal Government, APHIS/AC section for a description of animal care jobs, then contact your local government agencies to find out who is responsible for carrying out those duties where you live.

Resources: City/County jobs

See also: Association and Organization jobs.

Groups

1. The American Humane Association
63 Inverness Dr East, Englewood CO 80112-5117. Has a "Shelter Veterinarian Educational Program" for DVMS.
2. The Humane Society of the United States
2100 L St NW, Washington DC 20037
3. Association of Animal Shelter Veterinarians
See the current *AVMA Directory* for contact information. Has a quarterly newsletter.
4. National Animal Control Association
Johnnie W. Mays, Exec Director, PO Box 480851, Kansas City MO 64148-0851, 1-800-8286474 Fax 913-768-0607 naca@interserv.com
http://www.netplace.net/naca
Publishes a bimonthly magazine that includes advertisements for job openings for animal control veterinarians. Holds training conferences for animal control workers.

Articles

1. *Veterinarians serving US animal care and control facilities.* B Yoffe-Sharp. JAVMA 209 (10) 11/15/96 pp 1692-1696.
2. *Animal care and control center.* Dan Parmer. JAVMA 191(6) 9/15/87 pp 658-659.
3. *An idea whose time has come: Veterinarians in humane society administration.* Gary Patronek. JAVMA 202(6) 3/15/93 pp 862-864.

STATE JOBS

In general, state positions for veterinarians focus on public health, control of livestock disease, and zoonoses. Advancement to managerial and administrative positions is possible. The main employment opportunities are with the Public Health Department and the Department of Agriculture.

State Departments of Health are mainly concerned with human health. As all veterinarians know, this is directly related to animal health through the food supply and zoonotic disease. State Departments of Agriculture are mainly concerned with animal disease control. Since that can directly affect human health, there can be quite a bit of overlap among job duties. Job titles for veterinarians vary by state. Some states will put the Department of Health in charge of a certain area, whereas other states put their Department of Agriculture in charge of that very same area. Examples of this potential overlap include a variety of food programs such as milk or egg programs or organic foods certification. Although most job titles with the words "public health" in them are hired in the Public Health Department, there are exceptions. For example, Washington state's Department of Agriculture has a Food Safety and Public Health Division which hired a *Public Health Advisor* who is a DVM (although the DVM was not required for the position, the degree was considered to provide the necessary expertise).

Department of Public Health

Veterinarians have fantastic opportunities in various sections of State Departments of Health, which hire a wide variety of scientists.

As with Federal jobs, the best advice is this: take any job with the state that you can get, then you will find a wealth of other job opportunities that weren't obvious from the "outside." Also, once you're "in," you can educate others about the qualifications DVMS have that make them ideal for jobs they might not have been considered for in the past. Another tip: states with small budgets and low populations are more likely to hire DVMS for jobs with titles like *toxicologist* or *epidemiologist*—even if the applicant doesn't have a toxicology or an epidemiology degree—since these states rarely have the budget to hire a specialist. Once you've gotten experience, you can move on to a state with a larger budget, with "experience" on your resume. Jobs may focus on radiation safety, toxicology, epidemiology, and many more areas. People interested in focusing on the details of one aspect of their training might like this work. Others may take a job with a narrow focus as a springboard to other jobs.

Getting epidemiological training

Many city or state jobs require some knowledge of epidemiology or public health. It is possible to get an MPH in one year, a minimal time investment that may pay off handsomely.

You can also acquire new knowledge without "going back to school" in the traditional sense. Many accredited universities offer "distance learning" that allows you to take courses online or via correspondence. You can also join the military to have part or all of your education paid for. *See* "Going back to school" in Chapter 2 for more information.

EpiVet Net has list of short- and long-term online courses in epidemiology.
http://www.epiweb.massey.ac.nz/

Several states employ a S*tate Public Health Veterinarian* (PHV). There are 30 of these listed in the *AVMA Directory*; of those, most have a Masters or PhD degree. Because Public Health Departments focus on human health, the DVM's work will be in zoonotic and foodborne disease, but also may occasionally overlap into human disease issues. Veterinarians in environmental health may perform risk assessments of toxic sites or insecticide toxicity studies.

Salary varies considerably among states and by position. For instance, the salary for the state public health DVM is the lowest in Arizona ($36,000), averages about $55,000, and is highest in New York (around $96,000) (1996 figures).

Public Health Veterinarian

"I am not a bureaucrat—I really do hands on active public health work! I deal with hantavirus, plague, rabies, cat scratch disease, Simian B virus, brucellosis, tick-borne diseases, mosquito-borne diseases, rabies, more rabies, and any other vector-borne or zoonotic disease, including reptile-associated Salmonella. I do everything from case investigation and consultation, to field surveillance (collecting rodent blood for hanta, fleas for plague) to writing articles and guidelines, to lecturing and public speaking, to writing and defending legislative issues about rabies and zoonoses, to organizing and collaborating with universities or other organizations on projects that involve zoonotic disease issues. It is very diverse.

"I am a member of the *National Association of State Public Health Veterinarians* and sit on two committees there—the Rabies Compendium committee, and the coalition of public health veterinarians. The latter is a group of military, FDA, USDA, academic, state and local PH vets that discusses issues by teleconference. I travel around the state as needed, and to conferences out of state about twice a year. I stay current on worldwide outbreaks through an online group called *Promed*, and disseminate information to many state and local groups. As you can tell, I love my job, and am always happy to promote PH to veterinarians looking for alternatives. I am enrolled in a Masters in Public Health program, which is fairly essential to working in this field."—*Mira Leslie, State Public Health Veterinarian, AZ*

To apply

Look for job advertisements in each state's personnel division (the easiest way to find listings is to look on the state's Web site; otherwise, contact the department by telephone or mail). Apply for any job that involves the subjects you studied in veterinary school—and be ready to educate the hiring agency about how much you know. At least two of the DVMs interviewed for this section started by taking that approach in smaller states that were willing to hire veterinarians without advanced degrees. They've now moved on beyond their initial jobs to those that better serve their needs—but those first jobs got their feet in the door.

Openings for a State Public Health DVM are typically advertised in JAVMA and traditional veterinary-job resources. According to one incumbent, turnover is slow and is mostly due to retirement. However, a DVM living in a state without a PHV could take another Health Department position, and if the environment is supportive, perhaps create the PHV position (this has been done at least once in recent years).

Resources

(Note: See current AVMA *Directory* for updated listings)

Groups

1. *American Public Health Association.*
1015 15th St NW, Washington DC 20005; 202-789-5600.
2. *American Association of Public Health Veterinarians.*
c/o Dr. John Herbold, Univ of TX School of Public Health, 7703 Floyd Curl Dr, San Antonio TX 78284; 210-567-5930; herbold@uthscsa.edu
3. *National Association of State Public Health Veterinarians.*
Meets annually at the AVMA annual meeting.
c/o Dr. Kathleen Smith, Ohio Dept of Health, 246 N High St, Columbus OH 43266; 614-466-0283; ksmith@health.ohio.gov
or, Dr. Mary Grace Stobierski, MI Dept of Public Health, Disease Surveillance Section/DCD/BIDC; 3500 N Martin Luther King Jr Blvd, Lansing MI 48909, 517-335-8165
See the current AVMA *Directory* for current address and phone number.

Online

Food safety-related exercises for public health officials, focusing on the investigation of foodborne disease outbreaks, can be found on the "Food Safety CAI" site: http://sable.cvm.uiuc.edu/

STATE DEPARTMENT OF AGRICULTURE

Each state has a Department of Agriculture or similar agency. (e.g., Montana's Livestock Board, Louisiana's Livestock Sanitary Board, Nevada's Division of Agriculture).

Because each state has a different agricultural emphasis, jobs existing in one state may not exist in another. For instance, North Carolina employs a DVM as the S*tate Inspector of the National Poultry Improvement Plan,* a regulatory program to help ensure healthy poultry from egg to slaughter. (This person was a new graduate hired after doing a 1-year poultry internship.)

Management and supervisory positions

Many jobs for veterinarians exist within each state's Department of Agriculture. The most obvious are the state veterinarian and others who work under that person (*See* "Animal Disease Control," below). However, other positions are also available. Veterinarians have worked as Directors, Assistant Directors, and Commissioners in state Departments of Agriculture. The following description illustrates similar positions in other states.

The *Assistant Director of the Food Safety/Animal Health Division of the Washington State Department of Agriculture* is a veterinarian. Her experience included other state jobs (including working as a toxicologist in another state, and as a state public health advisor; *see* "jobs in public health," above). The Assistant Director is in charge of several programs, with a primary focus in public health: animal health (the state veterinarian's office); food safety (wholesalers and dairy farms); the egg program (from production to retail sale); and organic food certification. She supervises managers who run each of these programs; speaks to the legislature and to other groups; and performs administrative and managerial tasks.

Many management jobs such as this one are "exempt" positions—which means they're appointed or elected, and often are not advertised to the public. People with experience in other state jobs are thus more likely to hear about, and be considered for, management positions.

Assistant Director, Department of Agriculture

"I really enjoy public service, because I feel I'm making a bigger impact than I would working with individual animals in private practice."—*Candace Jacobs, Assistant Director, Washington State Department of Agriculture.*

Animal disease control

Animal disease control job titles and descriptions vary among states. *Below are job descriptions for some of the jobs available in Washington and California to give you a general idea of what's involved in these types of jobs.* Par for the course with government jobs, the "official descriptions" may be changed at any time. Nonetheless, in spite of "reorganizing" or changing of job titles, the essence of these jobs as described below is still accurate. Depending on the state, these job descriptions may overlap, be combined into one job, or be divided among jobs with different titles.

Every state has an *"official in charge of animal disease control,"* but the job title varies. In many states, that official is the *state veterinarian.* See the AVMA *Directory* for other titles; they range from "Administrator, Division of Animal Industries" (ID) to "Executive Secretary, Board of Animal Health" (MN) and "Chief, Bureau of Animal Industry" (IA).

The official in charge has several other DVMs working in the same office. These may include the assistant state veterinarian; state public health veterinarian; state meat inspector; veterinary medical officer; and animal health veterinarian. Entry-level jobs involve hands-on inspections, investigations, and travel; jobs higher up in the hierarchy are supervisory and desk positions.

Some states hire veterinarians for meat inspection; in other states, meat inspection is done by Federal veterinarians (*See* USDA—FSIS). To find out the case in your state, call the state veterinarian's office.

See the AVMA *Directory* under "government agencies" for addresses in your state, then write or call and ask for job descriptions for all jobs open to DVMS. Another place to look, especially for jobs other than those based in the state DVM's office, might be the State Department of Personnel (find on-line, or call your state capital's information).

State Veterinarian (WA)

The state veterinarian supervises and enforces laws relating to disease prevention, control, and eradication (especially in large animals), meat inspection, and all other matters relative to livestock diseases and their effect upon public health. The work includes assembling laboratory results, and evaluating data and classifying tests.

The state DVM is responsible for the interstate permit system; disease eradication programs (e.g., pseudorabies, TB); supervising farm inspections for the tissue antibiotic residue program; issuance of rendering plant licenses; submission of applications for Federal contracts for state public health programs; attendance at appropriate board and committee meetings (e.g., zoonoses committee, industry livestock groups, health committees, etc); and coordinating the state program with that of the USDA.

Daily work

The state DVM works out of an office in the state capital. This is primarily a desk position that involves delegating, supervising, and coordinating. About 25% of the time is spent attending or traveling to and from meetings. Two to three meetings per year are out of the state. Preparing budget documents, preparation for legislative sessions, and preparing planning documents take up about another 25% of the time. Phone time is about 5-10%.

Qualifications / Pay

This type of high-ranking position requires previous regulatory work in state or Federal Government. Pay range in WA state (1996) is $45,780 - 58,584. There are 11 automatic pay-increase steps (5% per step), with cost-of-living raises granted by the legislature. Benefits are good.

Assistant State Veterinarian (WA)

The responsibilities of this job include assisting the State DVM in all areas. The Assistant State DVM is the operational manager to whom all the field DVMs report directly, while the State Veterinarian is the administrative manager, whose job includes strategic planning, rule changes, overall policy matters, and interaction with client and stakeholder groups. The Assistant State DVM works out of the state office, with daily work similar to that of the state DVM.

Qualifications / Pay

Assistant State DVMs must have knowledge of the etiology, pathology and epidemiology of animal disease and toxicology; Federal and state laws and regulations pertaining to the control, eradication and transmission of the infectious livestock diseases within the state; and computer use for word processing, statistical analysis and spreadsheet operation. They must have the ability to work with owners and processors in inspection and control of livestock; plan and direct inspections throughout the state; develop proposed laws and rules pertaining to animal disease; work with veterinarians; supervise others; and write well. The position requires a DVM degree plus four years of large animal medicine experience, or two years of regulatory experience (e.g., Animal Health DVM).

The pay range (1996) is $41,460 to $53,100, with step increases and benefits.

Animal Health Veterinarian (WA)

The AHV is responsible for public health protection in one of four areas of the state. The AHV performs animal and herd examinations, conducts epidemiologic investigations, establishes and releases quarantines, investigates zoonotic diseases, and investigates animal welfare complaints. The AHV also acts as liaison between the state DVM and livestock groups; investigates and prepares cases for fines or prosecution; inspects, investigates, and licenses custom meat facilities (USDA-FSIS performs most other meat inspection); and investigates meat drug residue findings.

Daily work / Pros and cons

The WA state AHV spends most of the time doing field or epidemiologic investigative work. For example, if a drug residue problem is found, the AHV traces the animal to the farm of origin, contacts the producer, and conducts an on-farm interview to identify the potentials for residue introduction. About one day a week, on average, is spent doing paperwork or working on reports. The AHVs do all their own office work. They all work out of their homes, so their time is flexible. They file weekly time and project reports and adjust their schedules to a 40-hour week. The work involves lots of driving and working outdoors, no matter what the weather; they may be working with ranchers or farmers who are angry about having their premises quarantined or having a disease or drug residue problem.

Qualifications / Pay

The AHV must have knowledge of Federal and state laws and regulations pertaining to the control, eradication and transmission of the infectious livestock diseases within the state, and investigational procedures for judicial review and legal prosecution. The AHV must be able to work with owners and processors in inspection and control of livestock; plan and direct inspections in the area; work with veterinarians, livestock industry, media, and the public; and write well. The position requires a DVM and three years' experience in agricultural veterinary medicine. The pay range is $37,572 - $48,072 (1996) with step increases and benefits.

Veterinary Medical Officer—Animal Health (CA)

California's Division of Animal Industry in the Department of Food and Agriculture has three classes in the Veterinary Medical Officer, Animal Health series (VMO; VMO III ; and VMO IV).

There are VMOs and VMO IIIs in several regions of the state; the VMO IVs work in a district that comprises several regions, or they work on a statewide level on one particular disease. The VMOs perform the professional responsibilities of veterinarians working in the prevention, control, and eradication of livestock and poultry diseases. They investigate epizootic livestock and poultry diseases and disease outbreaks; recommend measures to prevent spread of epizootic diseases; plan effective methods of prevention and eradication of such diseases; consult with other agencies and institutions involved in related research; write reports and technical publications; and do other related work.

Daily work

The VMO is the entry/training level person who works under close supervision conducting routine veterinary tests; making veterinary inspections; learning the regulations, philosophy, and work of the agency; and gaining experience in laws, regulations, field procedures, epidemiology, diagnosis and handling of the public and industry in disease outbreak situations. Their work roughly corresponds to that of the WA state AHV, above.

The VMO III is the "journey level" person whose duties are to plan, organize, and coordinate veterinary work in the prevention, control, and eradication of livestock and poultry diseases in the region. They provide technical guidance and training to lower-level staff, act as district specialist in one or more diseases, and assist in the administration of the district. They provide technical assistance to local veterinarians and coordinate the activities of contract DVMs through field visits; evaluate the effectiveness of programs; determine the applicability of established procedures for disease prevention, control, and eradication; develop and recommend new practices and procedures; and prepare reports.

The VMO IV acts as a full supervisor of a district, or as a staff specialist with statewide responsibility for one or more diseases. Supervisor duties are to plan, organize, direct, and coordinate regulatory veterinary work in a district; develop and control the district budget; evaluate the effectiveness of district programs and recommend improvements; and train staff. Staff specialist duties are to plan and organize one or more major statewide disease programs; consult with and advise district DVMs; study unusual or exotic diseases; develop new or improved measures to control or eradicate diseases; and prepare scientific articles for publication.

Qualifications

All applicants must score at least 70% on an oral exam to be eligible; the highest scorer gets the job. Applications are not accepted on a promotional basis. The testing office accepts applications continuously and notifies job applicants as openings arise.

vmo jobs require a dvm degree and state license. The applicant must have detailed knowledge of food animal medicine, diseases and parasites, be able to speak and write effectively, and be willing to travel. vmo iii requirements are as the vmo's, plus experience in animal disease prevention and control that includes field work in livestock or poultry disease regulatory work. They must have knowledge of state and Federal laws pertaining to livestock and poultry diseases and necropsy procedures, and must be able to plan and direct the work of others. vmo iv requirements are as the vmo iii's, plus experience in animal disease, prevention, and control that includes regulatory work. They must have knowledge of public administration, personnel management, and supervision.

Veterinary Medical Officer—Meat Inspection

As with Animal Health, California's Meat Inspection vmos are classified as vmo i, ii, and iv. The levels of experience required are also similar to those described above. These are great jobs for people interested in pathology. For a description of the details of a meat inspection job, *see* Federal jobs, fsis.

Resources: State jobs

Groups

1. National Association of State Departments of Agriculture
1156 15th St NW Suite 1020, Washington DC 20005; 202-296-9680; NASDA@PATRIOT.NET http://www.nasda-hq.org/
2. National Assembly of Chief Livestock Health Officials
c/o Dr. Frank Rogers, PO Box 4389, Jackson MS 39296; 601-354-6089
3. National Association of State Meat and Food Inspector Directors
c/o Mr. Terry Burkhardt, PO Box 8911, Madison WI 53708; 608-224-4725

Online

Food safety-related exercises for public health officials, focusing on the investigation of foodborne disease outbreaks, can be found on the "Food Safety CAI" site: http://sable.cvm.uiuc.edu/

EXTENSION JOBS

The Cooperative State Research, Education and Extension Service (CREES or CSREES) is an education network based at 74 of the nation's land-grant universities, plus Tuskegee University. Land-grant universities have a trio of mandates: teaching, research and service (extension). CREES operates as a partnership of the Federal Government through the USDA and state and local governments. About 70% of the system's funding originates from state and local sources, with the rest from the Federal Government. (In your local phone book, extension agencies are listed under county government; in the AVMA *Directory*, they're listed under USDA; here, I've included them in the state/local government section, based on the amount of funding those governments provide and where you apply for these jobs.)

Extension agents work in most counties of each state. You have probably heard of the job of "Extension veterinarian," but veterinarians may also fill jobs titled "Extension agent" (recently changed to "Extension Educator"), where only part of their job is directly related to veterinary medicine.

County extension educator (agent)

Extension agents are basically information brokers with a broad range of duties. They provide educational and technical assistance in livestock and crop production, family life and community development. They may provide information about subjects such as home economics, making candy, sewing, growing apples, raising sheep, caring for horses, planting pasture or growing oats.

Extension personnel are responsible to the taxpayers in the community, so there must be a lot of taxpayers with a particular need (e.g., dairy farmers) to have a specialist for that need (dairy extension specialist). Thus if you want to work in a particular area (e.g., with horses), then you'll want to apply for an extension job in a county or state where the economy depends on that to some extent (e.g., Kentucky).

Daily work

A new extension agent may be asked to do a "community needs survey" to find out what needs exist and what programs are desired. The agent's job is then to deliver the information, by looking it up, teaching classes, finding volunteer teachers who are knowledgeable in the subject, or by giving out printed information. Organizing, writing, and distributing educational handouts on a variety of subjects is part of the job. Much of this work will be transferred to computers and distributed over the Internet in the future.

Extension educators respond to calls from community members, and find materials they need or a person to contact. They also conduct or organize classes on a variety of subjects. Collaborative relationships are established with county commissioners, the 4-H, the state university, schools, organizations, and agencies. The amount of administrative work varies, but is typically 15% of the job duties.

A typical winter day in northern states is spent indoors. Summer days include lots of outdoor work with 4-H activities. Extension agents may coordinate 4-H programs; tell people about the information they offer, then get it to them by phone or mail; write a newsletter; and organize meetings. They may telephone several people to find someone to write an article about food safety for their upcoming newsletter, or to find someone to give an educational talk about dairy herd management.

Most extension agents have assistants, who may include a secretary or 4-H program assistant. They also train local volunteers who train others (examples include master gardeners, master food safety advisors, clothing and textile advisors, livestock advisors, master weed advisors, or master dairy goat farmer (a subset of master livestock advisor)). The educator must recruit, screen, train, and counsel volunteers who help develop and implement these programs, and can recruit any people for any position where there is a need. Volunteers get something back, too: the master gardeners get free classes and materials from the university (which are brought to them), then they have to give back volunteer hours.

Volunteers may only give out advice sanctioned by the university—which tends to be traditional, chemical-based horticulture, but is gradually changing to allow for sustainable agriculture, long-term planning, integrated pest management, crop rotation, and organic farming.

Each state has county supervisors who supervise the extension educators. This would include a lot of administrative work. County supervisors are supervised by district coordinators.

Pros and cons

As an extension agent you'll still have contact with animals and animal owners, but without the need to take emergency calls or to run a business. Hours can be long, though. You'll be required to keep current on your medical knowledge, and you'll be able to learn more about other subjects, too. This is a very people-oriented job, and you'll be working with all ages, including school children.

Pay

Pay is adequate but not high ($25,000 and up, 1996), with good to excellent benefits. Advancement probably requires additional degrees beyond the DVM (e.g., in education or management). Some positions are on the university tenure track, with comparable advancement opportunities.

Extension Educator

"As an extension educator, I help people for free. This is a great change from private practice, where you have to charge for your services. I sometimes miss the direct animal contact, but I am helping people more directly now by educating them about their livestock."—*Susan Kerr, DVM PhD, Extension Educator, Klickitat County WA*

Qualifications

An agricultural background is necessary, and a background in education is helpful or required, depending on the position. The area's economic base will determine the amount of time spent using knowledge of livestock or horses versus working in areas like home economics, orchard or pasture management, or gardening. Those people with proficiency in many areas are most likely to be hired. Emphasis is put on people skills, computer and distance education skills, communications skills, and the subject matter directly pertinent to the specific opening. Teaching and administrative experience and experience working with the news media are desired. The extension agent must have effective speaking, writing, and listening skills; experience working with groups and individuals; and the capability to work independently or as a team member.

To apply

There is no central repository for extension jobs, which are advertised differently by each state. Potential sources of job announcements include the Web site of your state's land-grant university (which should have a page devoted to the extension service); the USDA Web page (there are hot links from the USDA Web page to the extension pages they know about—look under "state partners" at http://www.reeusda.gov); advertisements in the classified section of larger cities' newspapers; or your state's Extension Director, whose office is at the university and who may have job notices for other states, as well as yours. *Also see* the AVMA *Directory's* list of extension services by state.

Resources

See also: Teaching jobs.

Groups

American Association of Extension Veterinarians
Dr. Thomas J. Lane, Box 100136, Univ of FL, Gainesville FL 32610, 904-392-4700 ext 4024 (Or see this year's AVMA *Directory* for current listing.) There are also state organizations of extension agents. Contact the national organization to get the address of your state's group.

Job announcements and online resources

1. Your local extension service office is listed in the government section of your phone book—under "county," then under "cooperative extension." However, extension agents are hired by the state's land grant university; call there and ask for the extension office.
2. *The Chronicle of Higher Education* is a national weekly tabloid of educational jobs and opportunities. Includes meetings, seminars, workshops, and classified employment advertising. PO Box 1955, Marion OH 43306-4055. http://www.chronicle.com
3. *Cooperative State Research Education and Extension Service* (CREES) http://www.reeusda.gov/
Jobs http://www.reeusda.gov/new/hrd/novlist3.htm

CHAPTER 16

WORKING FOR THE FEDERAL GOVERNMENT—CIVILIAN JOBS

Federal jobs can be divided into two broad categories: the uniformed and civil services. Currently, about 2600 veterinarians work for the Federal Government, including the uniformed services/military; almost half of these are working for the Food Safety and Inspection service. Civilian jobs are scattered throughout the US, with the majority in Maryland, Iowa, Texas, Georgia, and Virginia.

It's interesting to note that graduates of certain veterinary schools are more likely to end up working for the Government. The following schools had 5 to 9% of their graduates working for the Federal Government in 1995 (other schools had less than 5%): Auburn, Colorado State, Iowa State, Kansas State, Ohio State, Texas A & M, and Tuskegee University.

Government "downsizing" and reorganization has caused some departments to create hiring freezes or eliminate certain positions. Nonetheless, there are still great opportunities for veterinarians in Government jobs.

Because the pay scale and approach to applications is the same for many jobs, we'll start with that general information before proceeding to specific Government agencies and the positions within them. Remember that the first "test" to see if you qualify for a government job is to be able to wade through this chapter. If you can do so, you're ready to read the even more stuffy government literature.

Federal agencies

The main US Federal agencies that employ veterinarians are:

USDA (US Dept of Agriculture) includes:
    APHIS (Animal and Plant Health Inspection Service) includes:
        CEAH (Centers for Epidemiology and Animal Health)
        CVB (Center for Veterinary Biologics)
    FSIS (Food Safety and Inspection Service)
    ARS (Agricultural Research Service)
    ORACBA (Office of Risk Assessment and Cost-Benefit Analysis)

HSS (US Dept of Health and Human Services) includes:
    PHS (Public Health Service)—includes:
        FDA (Food and Drug Administration) includes:
            CVM (Center for Veterinary Medicine)
        CDC (Centers For Disease Control and Prevention)
        NIH (National Institutes of Health)

Dept of the Interior—FWS (Fish and Wildlife Service)

Dept of Commerce—includes:
    NMML (National Marine Mammal Laboratory)
    NMFS (National Marine Fisheries Service)

To apply

Many Federal employees will tell you this: *The first step to take in investigating any civilian Federal job is to apply for one.* This does not obligate you in any way, but it will speed up the hiring process once you pursue that. There are two approaches to applying for Federal jobs:

1. Make a general application for veterinary jobs through the USDA-FSIS and USDA-APHIS.

2. Search the Federal job listings (either via the Internet or the automated phone lines, listed later), and apply for specific job openings with specific agencies.

The latter approach is recommended if you want to apply for jobs that are not listed as specifically for a "veterinarian," but for which DVMS may be well qualified (see list at right). Consider using both approaches and then making decisions based on the job offers you get. Federal jobs are highly competitive. The more announcements you bid on the better your chances.

Federal job series numbers

Each Federal job type is given a series number; for example, veterinary jobs are "series 701." That's useless information when it comes to job hunting, though, since jobs aren't organized that way (you can't just find a list of all "series X" jobs in one place, nor is one office responsible for each series). The series number is more for the hiring agency's convenience, to classify the job (that's why you should look beyond the "veterinary"—series 701— jobs; there are plenty of jobs out there that have been classified under other series numbers, but are ideal for DVMS). So the best thing to do is to ignore the series number and just look for the agency or, better yet, the type of job you want.

If you want a Federal job, you should consider accepting the most desirable one available, even though it may not be your first choice. By getting into the system, many other Federal positions will be open to you. Federal jobs are advertised in four categories: 1) only employees of the agency concerned may apply; 2) only employees of the department may apply; 3) all Government DVMS may apply and 4) any DVM may apply. The vast majority of job openings are in categories 1-3; until you are "in," you are seeing only a few of the potential job openings. Most DVMS start in field positions with APHIS (VS or AC, see descriptions below) or in meat inspection with FSIS. They then work their way through various other jobs according to their interests and to openings that become available.

Note: many job positions are labeled **"Veterinary Medical Officer"** (vmo). That title is used to apply to such a wide variety of jobs that it is almost meaningless. Also, in spite of the "officer" word, these aren't military jobs. So, look beyond the "vmo" for a true job description.

Here's what to do: Submit an application to 1) fsis 2) aphis and 3) the address on any specific job announcements that you find through your Federal job search (see details about each agency that follow). That approach will allow you to be considered for the largest number of job openings. Remember, you can always turn down a job offer, but you can't accept one that you never see.

Federal veterinarians may work in various agencies, in any of these fields:

Biological science	Microbiology
Pharmacology	Zoology
Physiology	Toxicology
Genetics	Fish and wildlife
Fishery biology	Wildlife biology
Food inspection	Veterinary Medicine
Public health	("Series 701")
Physical science	Health physics
Food technology	Educator/teaching
Technical writing	Consumer safety

Food compliance/regulation
Husbandry (animal scientist)
Health science (epidemiology)
Occupational safety and health (Biosafety officer)

Once your application is sent in, your eligibility is rated and you are placed on a list of people who are contacted as vacancies occur. You will have more potential job offers if you list a wide range of acceptable geographic areas in which you'd work, but you have the option of placing limits on both the location and the number of hours that you will work. Doing so will automatically mean that you are not notified of any jobs that don't meet your strict requirements, so be careful with the limits you set.

To apply for "veterinary" jobs in USDA-APHIS, contact:

USDA-APHIS, Field Servicing Office, Butler Square West, 100 N Sixth St, Minneapolis MN 55403; Vacancy recording: 612-370-2200; Real person: 612-370-2193; To get a fax back of all vacancies, forms, etc.: 1-800-585-7407. Vacancies are listed on their Web site, but you must still fill out and submit the forms. http://www.aphis.usda.gov/

The following office handles all Federal civilian "veterinary" job opportunities, except for USDA-APHIS:

USDA, FSIS Personnel Operations Branch—Recruitment Examining Section, Butler Square West, 100 N Sixth St, Minneapolis MN 55403, 800-370-3747 or 612-370-2000. Ask for Announcement No FSIS-701-1, which is a booklet that describes USDA jobs and includes application materials, and Announcement number FSIS-1863-1, "Food Inspector Competition Notice."

Applying to the FSIS (Food Safety and Inspection Service) does *not* mean you're applying only for meat inspection jobs. It *does* mean that you're applying for any job labeled "veterinary" (i.e., series 701)—and thus it excludes many jobs for which you may be qualified (public health official, technical information specialist, fish biologist, etc). Although this application will be used primarily to fill FSIS positions, other Federal agencies, such as the ARS, FDA, and the VA occasionally request names of eligible applicants. Your name will be referred on the basis of how well you meet their qualifications, and that observation depends on how thoroughly you describe your experience and knowledge when you fill out the application form—take your time!

To apply for jobs that don't specifically say "veterinarian"

Contact the individual agency, as described in the following sections. When considering a Government job, remember to look beyond jobs that require a DVM, to those that simply ask for someone with a science background, or someone with a Bachelor's degree that you hold (microbiology, biology, chemistry). Why get hung up on a title when you could find a job that pays just as well as other "veterinary" jobs, and uses as much of your knowledge? Think of your overall qualifications, not your degrees (you write well, have held supervisory positions, etc). When filling out your application, don't limit your notes to only medical and technical areas. Include your experience or classes you've taken in management, speaking, writing, and so on.

The easiest way to get an overview of all the jobs is to call the recorded job vacancy phone numbers, or go to the Federal Office of Personnel Management's (OPM's) Web site (see listings that follow). However, the OPM does not automatically list vacancies from agencies with direct-hire authority, so, to be thorough, you should check each agency's job announcements.

Pay

Government worker pay is rated on the "GS scale." There are 15 GS levels and a senior executive service; within each are several steps of advancement. Recent college graduates usually enter Federal service at grades GS-5 or GS-7. New DVM graduates with little experience start at GS-9 level ($28,912 in 1996); those with a year of experience or a superior academic record start at GS-11. Most positions for DVMs are at the GS-12 level ($45,939 to $59,725) and above.

Advancement to the next higher pay rate (step increase) can be achieved if job performance has been acceptable. In addition, Congress authorizes salary increases to keep Federal pay competitive with the private sector. Employees may also be promoted by meeting full performance requirements and qualification requirements, to the highest level in their specific career ladder. To get promoted beyond that requires a change to a different job with a different career ladder (e.g., from field to management positions).

In addition to pay, you get great benefits: paid vacation, sick leave, and holidays; health and life insurance options; and a retirement plan. Don't forget to include these in your calculations when comparing other jobs—benefits are expensive! You can get the current GS pay chart on the OPM (Office of Personnel Management) Web site or at any employment office. (*See* references at end of section).

Government cut-backs

The USDA recently announced changes in the organization of both the APHIS and the FSIS. FSIS expects to reduce headquarters and non-frontline positions by 20%, and to consolidate into a smaller number of offices. Similarly, APHIS will consolidate its offices into two regional hubs. The goal is "greater sharing of resources," but the result may be fewer administrative positions for DVMs. The effect on lower-level jobs (meat inspection, veterinary services field positions, and animal care facility inspection) remains to be seen.

Confused?

These entry-level positions will give you a great overview of all Government positions:
AVMA Congressional Fellowship. Working in Washington, DC for a year is a great way to see what other DVMs are doing working for the Government. (*See* Association jobs section.)
The Public Health Service Commissioned Corps is an all-officer organization that provides a variety of employment opportunities for health professionals and students. Officers are most likely to be assigned to the CDC, EPA, FDA, or NIH. (*See* Uniformed services section).
The Public Veterinary Practice Career Program hires DVMs who have little experience or background, and trains them to fill APHIS positions. (*See* PVPCP section, in this chapter.)

UNITED STATES DEPARTMENT OF AGRICULTURE (USDA)

Animal and Plant Health Inspection Service (APHIS)

There is a wide variety of opportunities for veterinarians who might like to work with APHIS. These jobs potentially include small animal, equine, food animal, or marine animal work;

hands-on animal work, or management and supervisory positions; and more.

APHIS veterinarians are most often initially hired as *Veterinary Medical Officers* (VMOS) in either *Veterinary Services* or *Animal Care* (two of APHIS' 9 divisions). However, there are other veterinary positions as well.

A huge number of potential jobs exist for veterinarians within the APHIS divisions. As with other Government agencies, APHIS' organization can change any time. However, the basic job descriptions will remain similar. Don't let the following list of descriptions limit your imagination. If you are interested in any of the divisions or units within APHIS, you may be able to find a job there (or work your way up to a position there). *See* the Resource list at the end of this chapter.

APHIS **duties are to:**

- Prevent spread of animal disease between states
- Keep foreign animal diseases out of the country
- Eradicate exotic diseases that enter the country
- Eradicate domestic diseases of human health significance or of economic significance
- Assure safety and potency of veterinary biologics (vaccines)
- Carry out congressional mandates of the Animal Welfare Act
- Maintain international personnel to enhance exports and collect information about animal health worldwide.

APHIS jobs may be located at the Washington, DC, headquarters; at quarantine facilities in Honolulu, Los Angeles, Miami and other sites; at the APHIS National Veterinary Services Laboratory in Ames IA; at the Animal Health Information Systems and National Animal Health Monitoring System in Ft Collins, CO; at one of the four APHIS regional headquarters; or at one of many state offices. Many APHIS DVMS are field-based and live in small towns. Others select a more mobile path that leads to a headquarters staff assignment in DC or MD. APHIS VS officers are stationed at border crossings and ports of entry. They also supervise privately owned bird-import facilities.

Preventing the spread of animal disease is a major part of APHIS veterinarians' work. Diseases of concern include bovine brucellosis and swine brucellosis; bovine tuberculosis; swine pseudorabies; and sheep and goat scrapie. Veterinarians working in import/export are concerned with those diseases as well as "foreign animal diseases," those that don't exist in the US.

To apply: Veterinary Service and Animal Care

All the APHIS jobs discussed in the following section require the same application process. See the introduction of this section for the APHIS application address. All AC and VS -VMOS are hired in the GS-701 series (that just means the veterinary series), with an entry level of GS 9-11; promotion to the GS-13 and higher levels is competitive but possible for VMOS with only a DVM degree (relocation is necessary for advancement).

Most VS- and AC-VMOS start out by doing field work, with their home as a base. Some enjoy this work as a long-term career. Others apply for advancement as jobs open up in regional offices. To advance, you must be willing to move and must sometimes apply for different positions, because you will not necessarily get promoted from your current position.

The easiest way to get either of these types of positions is to apply through APHIS' recruitment program called the Public Veterinary Practice Career Program (PVPCP; *see* below). Another route to a VS or AC job is to first get a job with FSIS and then apply for the VS or AC job while holding the FSIS position.

APHIS Public Veterinary Practice Career Program

APHIS' *Public Veterinary Practice Career Program* (PVPC) hires DVMS who have little experience or background, and trains them to fill VS or AC positions. APHIS uses this program as a way to recruit people for Veterinary Services. DVMS can apply directly for a job in VS or AC, or they may apply to the PVPC program. Since PVPC is a recruitment tool, someone not already working for the Government might find a job faster that way. This program also provides the necessary "1 year experience" required of many VS/AC positions. PVPC positions are temporary training positions located at one of several "duty stations" around the country. After completing the year, PVPC-VMOS can apply for a permanent position in VS or AC.

APHIS **Animal Care**

APHIS animal care (AC) is composed of field and staff VMOS and animal care inspectors. *Animal care VMOS* are responsible for enforcement of the Animal Welfare Act and the Horse Protection Act, which govern the humane care and use of certain animals. There are AC-VMOS in every state. Veterinarians concerned about animal welfare might be interested in this type of job.

The Animal Welfare Act protects from inhumane treatment and neglect certain warmblooded animals raised for commercial sale, used in research, transported commercially, or exhibited to the public, and requires that these animals be provided at least the minimum standards of care and treatment required by the regulations. The Horse Protection Act prohibits horses subjected to soring—a painful practice used to accentuate a horse's gait—from participating in exhibitions, sales, shows, or auctions.

Animal Care accomplishes its mission in several ways: educating regulated industries and the public about the Animal Welfare Act, the Horse Protection Act, and the governing standards and regulations; performing unannounced compliance inspections of all licensed or registered animal dealers, exhibitors, research facilities, and in-transit carriers; liaison and cooperation with other Federal, state, and foreign agencies and industry groups; and development of regulatory proposal and policy under the Animal Welfare and Horse Protection Acts.

Animal Care Headquarters, located in Riverdale, Maryland, consists of two staffs under the Deputy Administrator's office: Resource Management Support and Animal Care. Field operations for these two staffs are coordinated out of three regional offices in Annapolis, MD, Fort Worth, TX, and Sacramento, CA. (These are the places you'd work if you wanted to advance to a managerial or supervisory position one day.)

Daily work

AC VMOS inspect animal care facilities, including breeding kennels and research laboratories. Since the Animal Welfare act requires that every research lab have a veterinarian on staff, the AC-VMO's job requires a lot of tact (this is a veterinarian evaluating a veterinarian!). The VMO must address the issues of animal pain and suffering, and explore the need for each research project in relation to the way the animals are used. The VMOS ensure that proper anesthetics and analgesics are used to avoid animal suffering. They review such factors as water and food; heating and ventilation; sanitation; pest control; animal handling; and record keeping. The VMO also inspects horse shows, exhibitions, sales and auctions, to be sure that there are adequate facilities, crowd control, and proper horse handling. Other inspection sites vary from circuses to Christmas tree lots where live reindeer are displayed.

The AC VMO spends a lot of time driving around to facilities, then walking through the facility for the inspection. Each inspection must be recorded (writing skills). AC VMOS also participate in symposiums and seminars to educate people about animal welfare programs and inspections (speaking skills). If deficiencies are found, the VMO must educate the facility staff about how to correct the problems (communication and diplomacy skills). Each VMO may have licensed technicians working under his or her guidance (employee management skills).

AC VMOS work in every state. Many keep offices in their homes. Ongoing training is considered paid work time; attendance at veterinary CE meetings is often paid for as well. A Government vehicle is provided for the VMO's use. The work schedule is flexible.

The AC VMO must often deal with facility employees who view the VMO as an adversary; some are hostile. Occasional interactions with angry animal rights groups may arise. One drawback reported by an AC VMO is that Government work often requires that you do a less-than-perfect job. If you strictly enforce the laws, perhaps shutting down a facility, you create complaints (by the facility) and thus a headache for your supervisor (who takes it out on you). At the same time, you can't ignore problems. Thus, the best approach is to figure out how to tactfully educate facility staff such that changes are made without creating a fight. Change takes a long time, so those eager to correct problems quickly may feel frustrated.

Qualifications

Qualifications for the AC VMO include professional knowledge of veterinary medicine; an ability to diagnose lameness in horses; knowledge of a variety of animals, from laboratory mice to marine mammals (their social, behavioral, nutritional, and medical needs); knowledge of the Animal Welfare Act; and knowledge of the operations of research facilities, exhibitors, pet suppliers, and animal transporters.

Veterinary Services

Veterinary Services (VS) is the public health arm of the APHIS. VS VMOS work at protecting and improving animal health, quality, and productivity. Their work usually involves herd health preventive medicine and public health medicine. A wide array of jobs are available for DVMS. *VS is divided into four sections*, whose work overlaps at times:

- Brucellosis Eradication
- Emergency Programs
- Import/Export
- National Animal Health.

APHIS Veterinary Services: Support Staffs

At the Riverdale, MD, VS Headquarters, *Operational Support staffs* (which include DVMS) for each of the sections maintain liaison with the nation's commodity groups, coordinate intra- and inter-agency projects, resolve policy and regulatory issues, provide technical expertise, and manage National Animal Health programs. Within National Animal Health, there is a *senior staff* DVM assigned to each species. These positions do not involve a lot of direct animal contact. Several other veterinarians may work directly with the senior staff DVM.

Staff DVM

The *senior staff veterinarian* for each species acts as an interface between APHIS and special interest groups (e.g., American Association of Equine Practitioners, for horses; American Association of Bovine Practitioners, for cattle; etc). This position involves staff management and administrative duties; scientific reading; meeting with experts about various diseases; providing phone consultation for veterinarians and Government agencies (both the US and other countries); and providing technical support via telephone, written documents (e.g., booklets, letters), E-mail and other means. About 20% of the time is spent traveling.

The senior staff DVM must have specific knowledge of the particular species under his or her jurisdiction. For instance, the senior staff DVM for equine diseases was an equine practitioner with many years of experience working with world-class performance horses, and thus had knowledge of equine international travel and import/export requirements, various equine special interest groups, and so on. This person came directly to the supervisory position from private practice, rather than from within Government, because a person with the required experience could not be found within the agency at that time.

APHIS Veterinary Services: Emergency Services

VS emergency services works to keep the US free from foreign animal disease. Within VS, the Emergency Programs staff coordinates efforts to prepare for and respond to outbreaks of exotic animal diseases. They monitor foreign animal health and maintain an intensive surveillance system aimed at rapidly detecting and diagnosing outbreaks of exotic diseases in the US; provide laboratory support in determining if animals suspected of harboring foreign diseases are actually infected; and provide training to Federal and State veterinarians, animal health technicians, epidemiologists, port veterinarians, and others. When practicing veterinarians identify a possible incidence of foreign animal disease and report it to APHIS, Emergency Programs staffers work with them to make a definitive diagnosis. Through its computerized information system, Emergency Programs is able to access relevant literature about livestock and poultry diseases. Emergency Programs also maintains a lending library of more than 5,000 color slides (photographs of foreign animal diseases and VS-related subjects), and has a variety of instructional videotapes.

APHIS Veterinary Services: Import-Export

The vs *import-export section* regulates the importation of animals that enter the country through land ports along the borders with Mexico and Canada and through animal import or export centers in FL, NY, CA, and HI. Bird imports must enter through one of six vs-operated bird quarantine centers or through a privately owned, vs-supervised quarantine facility (the number of birds being imported has dropped significantly in recent years). vs also provides service to the aquaculture industry by issuing export health certificates for live fish and fish eggs exported to other countries.

Quarantine facility vs vmos work at all of these facilities. As an example, the Miami facility employs five veterinarians; three work "in the barn," and two perform more of the office work. Office work includes examining and endorsing health certificates, making sure that both the US and other countries' regulations are being met.

Quarantine station vmos meet the airplanes bringing in imported animals, or escort exported animals to their planes; supervise loading and unloading; take blood samples; and perform physical exams upon arrival and daily during the quarantine period. A wide variety of animals come through the station, including Olympic-quality horses, cattle, pigs, ostriches and vultures. Quarantine station vmos may inspect facilities that import animal products, or examine farms that are doing pre-export isolation.

The import-export jobs include lots of overtime work, since the vmo must be present when planes arrrive or take off. A background in mixed practice is ideal because of the knowledge of large animal diseases, vaccinations, and health certificate procedures.

APHIS Veterinary Services: National Animal Health Field Service

In each state, there are several *Field Service* vs vmos, whose work is often based out of their homes. vs vmos in field positions are assigned to specific geographic areas and must work with all species in their area. However, veterinarians who want to work with one particular species may be able to do so. Since you must work with whatever animals are in your area, you can limit your job search to areas where the species of interest is in high numbers. For instance, vs vmos in Iowa may see a lot of pigs, whereas those in Kentucky may see a lot of horses.

Field service: daily work

The vs vmo *field work* involves physical activity, including physical examination and evaluation of cattle and horses (e.g., climbing over gates, looking into trucks, crouching down to examine animals, transporting and setting up portable cattle chutes, performing and reading tests). The vmo works outdoors some of the time (regardless of weather) and may be exposed to contagious disease. Supervising employees (animal health technicians) is a part of the job, as is speaking (e.g., to livestock groups).

vs vmos travel locally to perform their duties. They go to farms and ranches that have disease problems to evaluate their operations and to devise solutions. Follow-up visits ensure that the local veterinarian is continuing with the proper procedures. Establishing and lifting quarantines are part of the job (this may create anger and pressure tactics from affected ranchers). Inspections of schools and restaurants may be necessary (e.g., to evaluate whether they are properly disposing of their garbage, not giving it away to someone to feed to their pigs). At times, they may be called to other states for short-term work (3-4 weeks) if, for instance, there is an outbreak of disease that requires additional help.

In addition to working with individual farms, the vs vmo conducts epidemiologic studies of diseases, evaluates their spread, and develops procedures for examining, diagnosing, and certifying the health of various animals (desk work). The vmo also evaluates animals and animal products for import and export. Every task requires paperwork documentation.

Field Service: Qualifications

The vs vmo field position requires a dvm degree and one year of experience performing similar duties (*see* pvpc, above). Driving is part of the job, but most travel does not involve an overnight stay (expect 1-5 nights per month). Experience with large animals or poultry is necessary, as is knowledge of domestic and foreign animal diseases. The vs vmo must be able to gather and assess data, to resolve conflicts, and to write and speak well.

International work

Short-term international positions: There are great opportunities for field service vs vmos to work internationally. Import of certain animals from other countries requires quarantine of those animals for designated periods in both the originating country as well as in the US. vmos have the opportunity to volunteer to go to these quarantine stations for short periods (30 to 90 days) to monitor animals waiting to be shipped to the US. These positions, in countries as diverse as Zimbabwe, China, and Bolivia, are announced regularly through Government mailings sent to vmos throughout the country.

Port veterinarian

States that border Canada and Mexico have *Port vs vmos* at border crossings that allow the import and export of animals. Port vmos are also stationed at airports that allow international shipments of animals (e.g., Seattle, Miami, Chicago, New York). These veterinarians may have some field service duties in addition to their port duties.

In many instances, vs employees operate under state authorities in inspecting, quarantining, and regulating livestock and poultry (*See* "State jobs" section.)

Port vmo: Daily work

Port vmos endorse export papers, randomly inspect animals crossing the border, and in their "spare" time, conduct field service tasks (although the port work takes priority). Although these duties overlap, that doesn't create longer work hours. The port vmo may be far removed from his or her "boss," which allows for autonomy and creates a fairly low-pressure job. However, it is important to keep vigilant and not "slack off" after seeing lots of healthy animals come through the port; the vmo must always keep an eye out for signs of disease, mismarking of animals, and other problems. The work pace picks up when a problem is spotted.

Epidemiologist

Veterinary Services jobs also include *area and regional epidemiologists*. The position may focus on one species (e.g., "regional poultry specialist.") The job may require the ability to apply epidemiologic principles and to conduct epidemiologic studies; skill in applying regulatory guidelines and in communicating with others; and ability to perform statistical and epidemiologic analyses.

Epidemiologist: Daily work

The vs *epidemiologist* meets with industry groups to discuss disease control programs; plans and implements animal health monitoring and disease surveillance programs; and cooperates with nearby states in these endeavors. About 30% of the work time is spent traveling.

The *regional epidemiologist* vmo coordinates and conducts epidemiologic studies; develops and recommends methods and procedures dealing with disease spread; forecasts levels and location of disease development; develops scientific papers on new and improved disease detection and diagnosis; and meets with industry groups to promote compliance with disease eradication and control programs.

The *area epidemiologist* vmo has area-wide responsibility for planning, developing, and operating the epidemiologic delivery system. Duties include data analysis, risk assessment, coordinating with nearby states on difficult or unusual cases, forecasting disease incidence, and establishing budget and work plans accordingly.

Epidemiologist: Qualifications

Epidemiologist positions do *not* necessarily require an advanced degree in epidemiology, but they do require appropriate experience (often gained in other vs jobs, or by taking courses in epidemiology and statistics).

Area Veterinarian

There is also a vs *Federal Area Veterinarian-in-Charge* in most, but not all, states. vs field operations are coordinated by *Regional Directors* who operate out of offices in NY, FL, TX, and CO, and who report to the vs Deputy Administrator.

VS Science and technical units

The scientific and technical units of vs are:
* The *Centers for Epidemiology and Animal Health* (CEAH), in CO.
* The *Center for Veterinary Biologics* (CVB), in MD, IA, and NY.

Together they implement the provisions of the Virus-Serum Toxin Act to assure that safe and effective veterinary biologics are available—including those used by the aquaculture industry. Veterinarians may work in any of these units. For instance, a veterinarian working in the Veterinary Biologics section reviews and licenses veterinary vaccines and diagnostic test kits.

CEAH

The Centers for Epidemiology and Animal Health (CEAH) provides information and technical services for animal health and other agricultural interests to ensure a safe and economical supply of food and agricultural products.

Three Centers work together to accomplish the CEAH Mission. Veterinarians are employed in all these centers.
* The Center for Animal Disease Information and Analysis
* The Center for Animal Health Monitoring
* The Center for Emerging Issues.

CADIA

The Center for Animal Disease Information and Analysis (CADIA) collects, manages, analyzes, and disseminates information critical to vs programs and other APHIS initiatives. The bulk of their work falls under the broad category of information analysis. This includes risk analysis, epidemiological analysis, agricultural economic analysis, geographic information systems and geospatial analysis. They also train animal and plant health officers in these skills.

CAHMS / NAHMS

The Center for Animal Health Monitoring delivers timely, factual information and knowledge about interactions among animal health, welfare, production, product wholesomeness, and the environment. One of its activities is gathering information on the state of animal health in the United States through the vs *National Animal Health Monitoring System* (*NAHMS*). This program's goal is to provide statistically sound data concerning U.S. livestock and poultry. NAHMS conducts national studies to gather data and generate descriptive statistics and compiles statistics and information from data collected by other industry sources.

CEI

The Center for Emerging Issues (CEI) explores and assesses, with a view to the future, animal health and other agricultural issues in order to facilitate informed decision-making. The activities of CEI identify and use data and information from multiple sources to provide epidemiologic and economic assessments of present and emerging animal health-related issues. Such analytical projects are typically time-critical, and focus on specific issues that affect broad geographic areas and multiple industries. The CEI multidisciplinary team includes veterinarians, economists, statisticians, and epidemiologists.

Information technology

The *Information Technology Service*, whose mission is to strategically acquire and use information resources to improve the quality, timeliness, and cost-effectiveness of APHIS' service delivery to the customers, works closely with the above three centers.

Other APHIS jobs

Teaching or supervising positions are also available within APHIS. One veterinarian who had a teaching background became an "Education development specialist" and trained APHIS personnel involved with animals; she also helped supervise the PVPC program (discussed above).

Another job involves supervision of APHIS' Risk Analysis Systems Unit, which was organized to develop methods for assessing risks to US agriculture from imported diseases or pests.

There are a small number of *jobs overseas* with the Foreign Service; openings are limited. As with other international jobs, fluency in another language is important. The International staff help countries train their own animal health care workers or recommend programs to improve food animal health and productivity. (Short-term international positions are available for field service VMOS—see above.)

Food Safety and Inspection Service (FSIS)

The FSIS has permanent positions for veterinarians as food safety inspectors. These positions are a good stepping stone to other Government jobs (and some people even like the work without that motive!). Veterinarians are hired by FSIS as Veterinary Medical Officers (VMOS), or meat inspectors. The VMO is responsible for antemortem and postmortem inspection of livestock and poultry, and for making sure that plants and facilities meet Federal standards of cleanliness. People who like pathology may enjoy FSIS jobs.

This organization's duties are to ensure the wholesomeness of food and assure the safety of red meat and poultry sold in interstate commerce. Some states have their own meat inspection services, whereas others depend solely on FSIS. Veterinarian FSIS inspectors are in a supervisory position, with non-veterinarian inspectors doing the routine on-line inspections. The job is physically demanding, and is in a noisy, wet environment.

FSIS officers work in privately owned plants, where they examine live animals and carcasses after slaughter, as well as inspect facilities and make sure labeling is properly done. Some inspect only processed products (frozen dinners, canned goods, etc.); others inspect only carcasses; and others inspect both. Sanitary inspections of the plant and antemortem inspections (checking live animals before they go into the slaughter area) are part of the job. The VMO may work at very small or very large plants, with a few or many assistants. Hours may be long, and there may be night on-call duty (especially with larger plants that run around the clock).

The VMO is the "inspector in charge" who supervises several on-line inspectors. When a questionable live animal (antemortem inspection), carcass or organ (postmortem inspection) is found, the VMO is called to make a final judgement. Non-DVM inspectors are allowed to condemn individual organs, but the VMO must usually make the decision to condemn an entire carcass. Every decision must be documented with lots of paperwork. Some plants take in more questionable animals than others; at those plants, the VMO inspector has a lot more work to do and ends up spending overtime doing the necessary paperwork. VMOS are also responsible for doing drug residue checks. Any positives are traced back to the producer.

There are also "relief" jobs as FSIS VMOS. These are regular, full-time (sometimes overtime!) positions. The reliever is assigned a duty station in one city but works as a fill-in at plants where there is a vacancy or the regular veterinarian is sick or on vacation. These VMOS cannot specify how many days they want to work, but the income is good. One advantage for these VMOS is that they build up their resumes with a variety of experiences—from large plants to small ones, and working with a variety of animals and animal products. Usually the relief jobs are within a designated geographic area.

Qualifications

You must be physically fit (able to lift and carry 15-44 lb; able to stand/walk for hours at a time) and have good vision (including color—25% or more error rate on the approved color plate test is disqualifying).

Job offers are based on your eligibility (determined by the qualifications you list in your application) and the geographic limits that you indicate. Once employed, you can request transfer to another area; moves are likely to take two or more years (that's for transfers to another area, but still working as a food safety officer).

A VMO needs only a DVM degree. The USDA-FSIS hires 50-75 new veterinarians annually. Veterinarians receive on-the-job and classroom training. After completing a 1-year probationary period, they progress to the next GS level.

Further progression depends on your job performance and geographic mobility. By taking courses or volunteering for various committees, you can expand your knowledge into different areas. Once you become proficient at your job, you can advance to a teaching or supervisory position. FSIS VMOS are paid at the GS-12 level; you can advance to a "circuit supervisor" at GS-13, then to an "area/district supervisor," and on to a "regional director." Each level supervises the one beneath; these jobs require management skills, paperwork and travel. For example, the circuit supervisors keep an office in the home (although they are assigned a "duty station"), and spend much of their time driving to different plants for inspection.

Alternative routes to advancement are to move to Washington DC to take a job with office experience, then use that experience to help get a job nearer your preferred location; or to take on a teaching position, which can be located in a variety of areas.

Poultry plant inspector

"I derive a great deal of satisfaction from a neat, clean environment. Inspecting poultry plants seemed to suit this part of my personality and even reward it with a paycheck and the pleasure of protecting people's health."—*Dr. Barbara Soderstrom, in* Women in Veterinary Medicine: Profiles of Success, *Iowa State University Press 1991.*

Pros and cons

This job requires working at least six days a week in physically demanding environments. However, you do get overtime pay. VMOs don't work for the plant itself (they work for the Government), but they are working *in* the plant—thus they can be viewed as the "bad guy." New VMOs may be viewed with suspicion and have their judgement questioned. Taking a firm and consistent approach to every case is the key to developing respect. Food inspection includes viewing (over time) a large number of diseased organs, which can be fascinating for anyone interested in pathology.

To apply

See the introduction to this chapter for application address.

Resources

American Association of Food Hygiene Veterinarians
4910 Magdalene Ct, Annandale VA 22003-4363
The "Food Safety CAI" Web site contains "Simulated Antemortem and Postmortem Inspection" lessons. http://sable.cvm.uiuc.edu/

Agricultural Research Service (ARS)

The ARS has jobs for veterinarians in the area of animal disease research—the diseases and parasites of livestock, poultry and fur-bearing animals. Most veterinarians working with the ARS are researchers with additional degrees. However, the ARS does employ several veterinarians ("Veterinary Medical Officers," or VMOS) for clinical work. These DVMS maintain the health of research animals (dairy and beef cattle, sheep, swine, lab animals, some cats). They perform experimental surgery, such as installing rumen fistulas or placing catheters in blood vessels. They are responsible for routine health care such as treatment of mastitis, metritis, and other common disorders seen in practice. On-call duty is expected, but there are few emergencies.

ARS VMOS supervise one or more technicians, and attend various committee meetings. They work varying amounts of time with a variety of researchers (who may be easy or difficult to get along with), depending on the particular study, animals used and the care needed.

Openings are advertised in Government listings and in the *Journal of the AVMA*. Turnover is low so openings are rare. Some ARS openings are filled through USDA-FSIS (*see* "To apply" in general discussion of Federal jobs, above).

Resources

ARS Agricultural Research Service, Personnel Operations Branch
Bldg 003, BARC-West, Beltsville MD 20705;
http://sun.ars-grin.gov/~dbmuke/test/barc.html
or
ARS Agricultural Research Service, Personnel Operations Branch
6305 Ivy Ln Rm 101, Greenbelt MD 20770; 301-344-1124; 344-8506;
vacancy recording 301-344-2288
National Animal Disease Center, PO Box 70, Ames IA 50010, 515-239-8201

The Office of Risk Assessment and Cost-benefit Analysis (ORACBA)

This office began operations in 1995; its role is to ensure that major regulations proposed by the USDA are based on sound scientific and economic analysis. A "major regulation" is one that has an annual economic impact of at least $100 million and concerns human health or safety, or the environment.

ORACBA is responsible for making sure that USDA agencies proposing major new regulations conduct the required analysis. It provides guidance and technical assistance. The current Director of ORACBA is a veterinarian who holds a DVM and PhD, and whose background included a series of jobs within the USDA-APHIS, from Veterinary Services (VS) through supervisory positions. Although her job is unique within the Federal Government, Congress has publicly stated that there may be more such offices created at other agencies.

ORACBA **Director**

"I was fortunate to serve in APHIS, for they strongly encouraged continuing education and made many opportunities available. The biggest benefit of all is the fact that I love my job. It requires all my academic training, my continuing education learning and daily striving to learn even more. It gives me opportunities to interact with some of the best and brightest scientists and veterinarians in the USDA, in the Federal Government, and in the world. What more could one want?" —*Dr. Alwynelle Ahl, Director of ORACBA, 1997.*

Key functions of ORACBA include education and training (a seminar series informs agencies about risk assessment); coordination (help agencies identify resources, information and methods supporting their risk assessments); guidance (technical and analytical support to USDA agencies as requested); regulatory review (coordinate peer review of proposed major regulations); and risk information (assist in the development of risk assessment information services in USDA).

DEPARTMENT OF HEALTH AND HUMAN SERVICES (DHHS) PUBLIC HEALTH SERVICE (PHS)

The PHS has eight agencies, with three of interest to veterinarians:

- The Food and Drug Administration (FDA), which includes the Center for Veterinary Medicine (CVM)
- The Centers for Disease Control and Prevention (CDC)
- The National Institutes of Health (NIH)

Health professionals employed by the PHS are in one of two systems: the civil service system, or the PHS Commissioned Corps (*see* Military section). Begin your search with the following Web sites, then see the specific information for each agency.

DHHS Job Vacancies http://phs.os.dhhs.gov/psc/hrs/dhhsjobs.txt
DHHS links to HHS Agency Web pages http://www.os.dhhs.gov/progorg/

Food and Drug Administration (FDA)

The FDA has a large number of divisions that may hire DVMs. Some work under the VMO title, but others work as biologists or other scientists. Jobs within the FDA that a DVM might qualify for include veterinary medical officer (VMO); biologist; chemist; consumer safety officer; microbiologist; pharmacologist; toxicologist; or pathologist.

The FDA approves and regulates drugs and medical devices designed to prevent, control, manage or eradicate disease, and protects consumers from unsafe foods, cosmetics, drugs, and radiological products. They regulate the manufacture, import, transport, storage and sale of these products. The FDA's Office of Operations includes several Centers of interest to veterinarians:

- Center for Biologics Evaluation and Research
- Center for Devices and Radiological Health
- Center for Drug Evaluation and Research
- Center for Food Safety and Applied Nutrition
- Center for Veterinary Medicine
- National Center for Toxicological Research
- Office of Orphan Products Development
- Office of Regulatory Affairs

Most FDA jobs for veterinarians are with the CVM at the Maryland headquarters. However, jobs are also scattered throughout the country (the FDA has 6 regional offices, 21 district offices, and over 130 resident posts) and among all the Centers.

FDA *Center for Veterinary Medicine (CVM)*

The CVM is divided into four "offices." Each office consists of many divisions. Veterinarians work in all of these areas.

- Management
- Pre-marketing
- Post-marketing
- Research

Management

The *management staff* is responsible for overseeing the day-to-day operation of the Center. They oversee the setting and implementation of its goals and direction, manage personnel and the budget, and disseminate information.

Pre-marketing

The *pre-marketing staff* determines whether or not a drug should be approved for marketing (this ties in with industry jobs in product development; *see* Industry). The Office of New Animal Drug Evaluation is responsible for reviewing information submitted by drug sponsors who wish to obtain approval to manufacture and sell animal drugs. A new animal drug is deemed unsafe unless there is an approved new animal drug application. Virtually all animal drugs are "new animal drugs" within the meaning of the term in the Federal Food, Drug, and Cosmetic Act. Before a new animal drug may receive FDA approval, it must be clinically tested for effectiveness and safety. If a product is intended for use in a food-producing animal, it must also be tested for safety to human consumers, and the edible animal products must be free of unsafe drug residues. The sponsor must also develop analytical methods to detect and measure drug residues in edible animal products. It is the responsibility of the drug sponsor (the individual or firm seeking FDA approval of the drug product) to conduct the necessary tests.

Pre-marketing reviewers study data submitted by drug sponsors to determine if the data are adequate to support a drug's approval for marketing. One example of a pre-marketing Division is that of of therapeutic drugs for nonfood animals, which is divided into two teams (companion and wildlife drugs team, and antimicrobial drugs team). Veterinarians work for both of those teams. Another Division is that of therapeutic drugs for food animals.

New Animal Drug Application sponsors usually include university researchers, contract researchers, private practitioners, drug manufacturers, and/or feed or food manufacturers in their protocols. The activities of the investigators are monitored through the FDA's bioresearch monitoring program. Their data generation processes are validated through on-site inspections by FDA field personnel. Reports covering laboratory practices relating to toxicology and safety research, and the functions of clinical investigators and sponsors are forwarded to CVM for evaluation.

Post-marketing

The *post-marketing staff* monitor marketed animal drugs, food additives, and devices to assure continuing safety and effectiveness. They also process legal cases brought against violators by the Center. They work in cooperation with the FDA Field Offices, monitoring marketed animal drugs, food additives, and veterinary devices to assure their safety and effectiveness. This regulatory responsibility is carried out by scientists and by investigators and analysts around the country. One activity is the overseeing of medicated animal feeds. Another involves monitoring drugs used in food and non-food animals, and providing scientific expertise for legal cases. In addition, information is prepared by this group for dissemination to the public and regulated industry in an effort to encourage voluntary compliance with the laws and regulations enforced by FDA.

The FDA conducts regulatory followup on producers that have had tissue residue violations as reported by the FSIS. (The states usually conduct investigations on violations caused by first-time violators; FDA focuses its resources on repeat offenders.) The FDA also enforces the Pasteurized Milk Ordinance.

Research

The *research staff* conducts studies to aid CVM scientists in the review and decision-making processes. They conduct their own research and coordinate outside research grants and contracts; develop and validate procedures for analyzing drugs, additives, and contaminants in animal tissues and food; investigate the absorption, distribution, metabolism, and excretion of drugs, feed additives, and contaminants in food animals; determine the safety and efficacy of diagnostic agents and devices for animal use; and investigate interactions between diet and drugs in food producing animals.

Sample job announcement: FDA-CVM

Veterinary Medical Officer (VMO), GS-12, serving in the Rockville, MD Division of Therapeutic Drugs for Food Animals with responsibility for determining the safety and efficacy of new animal drugs. Reviews and interprets applications and scientific investigations regarding New Animal Drug Applications and Investigational New Animal Drugs, making sure they contain the necessary information and are approvable. Discusses the progress of applications with sponsors and prepares correspondence describing any deficiencies. Evaluates proposed labeling of new drugs. Integrates conclusions of consulting scientists into a comprehensive review. Requires DVM, 1 year of experience in clinical food animal medicine, writing and speaking skills, and ability to review and evaluate data. GS-12 $45,939 to $59,725.

To apply

The FDA has established an automated vacancy announcement system to inform individuals of current headquarters job openings and some field vacancies. The information lines are updated weekly. Some FDA jobs for DVMs are filled through the USDA-FSIS (*See* general discussion about applying for Federal jobs at the beginning of this chapter.)

Food and Drug Administration 5600 Fishers Lane, Rockville MD 20857 (Ask for the address of the Federal Regional Personnel Office nearest you.) Vacancy recording 301-443-1969; http://www.fda.gov FDA job opportunities: http://www.fda.gov/opacom/morechoices/vacancy/jobs.htm

FDA *Center for Veterinary Medicine*, 7500 Standish Place, Rockville MD 20855; Vacancy recording 301-594-1740; http://www.cvm.fda.gov/ FDA-CVM job announcements:
http://www.cvm.fda.gov/fda/infores/jobs/recruit.html
Center for Drug Evaluation and Research job announcements:
http://www.fda.gov/cder/career.htm

Centers for Disease Control and Prevention (CDC)

The Centers for Disease Control and Prevention, with headquarters in Atlanta, GA, works in such areas as prevention of infectious and chronic diseases, environmental health, occupational safety, international health, epidemiologic and laboratory research, data analysis, information management, and health promotion.

Most DVMs working at the CDC have additional degrees beyond their DVMs. However, there are a few opportunities for DVMs. Veterinarians who work for the PHS Commissioned Corps (*see* "Military jobs") may be assigned to work with the CDC. Other DVMs working for different Government agencies may be temporarily hired by the CDC.

The AVMA *Directory* has a listing of the CDC offices and the veterinarians employed at each, including the degrees they hold. This listing is somewhat deceptive if you consider the apparent number of "only DVMs" listed. Further investigation reveals that they have extensive experience in their fields; many are actually hired by agencies other than the CDC, but nonetheless work in the CDC. This confusing situation is best understood by talking to several different CDC veterinarians. The conclusion is the same, though: DVMs who are directly hired by the CDC have additional degrees (e.g., MPH) or board certification in laboratory animal medicine. (A CDC employee points out that an MPH can be obtained in 1 year.)

To apply

CDC Job Information Center/Announcement Postings:
Koger Center-Stanford Building, 2960 Brandywine Road, Atlanta, GA (770) 488-1725; CDC, Human Resources Management Office, 4770 Buford Highway, MS K-05, Atlanta, GA 30341-3724
recr@opshrmo.em.cdc.gov http://www.cdc.gov
24-hr Jobline—recorded message updated weekly (404) 332-4577
Job listings are posted on http://www.cdc.gov

Applications for specific vacancies can be sent to
Employment Information Service, CDC; Mail Stop K05, 4770 Buford
Highway, Atlanta, GA 30341-3724

CDC *Training and fellowships*

The CDC's *Epidemic Intelligence Service* is a 2-year post-graduate program of on-the-job epidemiology and statistics training for health professionals (physicians, dentists, and veterinarians). Veterinarians must also have a Masters of Public
Health to be eligible. Many of the veterinarians working with
the CDC were hired after going through this program.

A 2-year CDC *Public Health Informatics Fellowship* is available with the CDC. The fellowship requires some experience in
public health (which most veterinarians have to some degree
upon leaving school) as well as experience (or training) in
computers. Fellowship participants will be trained both in
informatics and in public health. This experience will help
equip them to guide the development, evaluation, and implementation of new public health surveillance and information
systems, as well as the adaptation and support of existing
ones. Fellows will be assigned to project teams involved in
both research and development of informatics systems as well
as concepts crucial to the support of CDC's mission of preventing disease and injury. Fellows who have completed their
training within the past three years are preferred. A monthly
stipend will be paid based on qualifications (ranges from
$2,405 to $3,600).

To apply

Postgraduate Research Program-CDC; Education and Training Division;
Oak Ridge Institute for Science and Education. P.O. Box 117, Oak Ridge,
TN 37831-0117, (423) 576-8503
CDC Contact: Div. of Public Health Surveillance and Informatics
Epidemiology Program Office, CDC; MS C-08; 1600 Clifton Road NE,
Atlanta, GA 30333, 404-639-3761; soib@epo.em.cdc.gov

National Institutes of Health (NIH)

The National Institutes of Health comprises 22 distinct institutes, centers and divisions and is headquartered in Bethesda,
Maryland. The NIH's mission is to supervise, fund and conduct research that produces new knowledge about disease

and disability in human beings. NIH research is oriented toward the prevention, diagnosis, and treatment of disease, and NIH-sponsored research discoveries have led to cures and therapies for afflictions ranging from cancer to schizophrenia.

Although most of the NIH's budget is spent on extramural research conducted throughout the United States, about 11% of the budget is spent on intramural research conducted at the NIH. The NIH's branches, any of which may have positions of interest to DVMS, include:

- National Cancer Institute
- National Institute of Environmental Health Sciences
- National Library of Medicine
- Office of Alternative Medicine
- Office of Disease Prevention

To apply

For veterinary positions within the NIH, apply through the USDA-FSIS (that is, for series 701 jobs—*see* explanation in chapter introduction). Many positions are also filled through the Commissioned Corps (*see* Military section). For other jobs (science, lab animal research, and epidemiology), contact:
NIH Recruitment and Employee Benefits Branch, Bldg 31, Rm B-3, C 15, Bethesda, MD 20892, 301-496-2403

The NIH Web site has a Resource Guide that lists the address, phone and fax numbers, and E-mail address of the directors and legislative liaisons of each of the NIH's component institutes and offices.
http://www.nih.gov or
http://www.aamc.org/research/adhocgp/aboutnih.htm

FISH AND WILDLIFE SERVICE (FWS)

The FWS is a bureau within the Department of the Interior. Its mission is to conserve, protect, and enhance fish and wildlife and their habitats for the continuing benefit of the American people. Its major responsibilities are migratory birds, endangered species, certain marine mammals, fish, the National Wildlife Refuge System, wetlands, conserving habitat, and environmental contaminants. The FWS is divided into 7 geographic regions, with its headquarters in Arlington, Virginia. The FWS employs a small number of veterinarians.

To apply

General Fish and Wildlife job information:
National Wildlife Health Lab, 6006 Schroeder Rd, Madison WI 53711; 608-271-4640; http://www.doi.gov/
For information on careers:
http://www.fws.gov/./who/careers.html
For job openings with the Service see:
http://info.er.usgs.gov/doi/avads/index.html
http://www.doi.gov/doi_empl.html

NATIONAL MARINE MAMMAL LABORATORY (NMML) AND NATIONAL MARINE FISHERIES SERVICE (NMFS)

These agencies have a few job openings related to research or fish inspection; all are under the National Oceanic and Atmospheric Administration. Contact the appropriate regional office of the NOAA Administrative Support Center, Personnel Division:

Western, RAS/WC2; 7600 Sand Point Way NE, BIN C15700; Seattle WA 98115-0070; 206-526-6294
Mountain, RAS/WC2; 325 Broadway, Boulder CO 80303; 303-497-6292
Central, RAS/CC2; Federal Bldg Rm 1740, 601 E 12th St, Kansas City MO 64106; 816-426-5016
Eastern, RAS/EC2; 200 World Trade Ctr, Norfolk VA 23510; 804-441-6516

US AGENCY FOR INTERNATIONAL DEVELOPMENT (USAID)

USAID is a Federal Government agency, established in 1961 by President John F. Kennedy, that conducts foreign economic assistance and humanitarian aid missions to advance US economic and political interests overseas. Missions have the authority to hire contractors and interns to meet requirements of their staff operations. Non-US citizens and US citizens may apply for contract positions, and citizens may apply for contract and intern positions. The agency does not employ veterinarians for direct-hire positions.

To apply

Contact each of the USAID Missions directly for information. A list is found on their Web site, or write USAID and ask for the list.

1. US Agency for International Development, Office of Human Resources, Recruitment Unit; Room 671 SA-36 Washington, DC 20523-3609, or 1550 Wilson Boulevard, Room 658A SA-36, Washington, D.C. 20523-3607. Fax (703) 302-4095; Information Hotline and Fax-On-Demand (703) 302-4128; Agricultural enterprises, USAID 202-663-2529 http://www.usaid.gov/

2. USAID contract employment opportunities are listed in the *Commerce Business Daily*. For subscription call (202) 512-1800 and give the Government Printing Office Stock Number 703-013-000007, List ID "COBD".

3. The *Current Technical Services Contracts and Grants Book* (W-443 better known as the Yellow Book) has contract award information for subcontracting opportunities. For copies, call the Office of Procurement, Contract Information Management System Staff 703-875-1091.

4. The USAID Bureau for Humanitarian Response (BHR), Office of US Foreign Disaster Assistance (OFDA), has positions for US citizens only. Experience in overseas civil strife is required for domestic and overseas positions. Fax your application to (202) 647-5269 or mail to USAID/BHR/OFDA, Washington, D.C., 20523-0008.

USAID *Fellowships for veterinarians*

The US Agency for International Development offers 1-year *Science and Engineering Diplomacy Fellowships* (renewable for a second year) for professionals interested in international work. One veterinarian is chosen each year. These fellowships, like the AVMA Congressional Fellowships (*See* "Association work,") are sponsored by the American Association for the Advancement of Science (AAAS). The program emphasizes networking among a variety of professionals to solve problems in another country; the specific focus is up to the fellow to determine (guidance is provided). The purpose of bringing in professionals such as DVMs is to augment the general nature of the personnel at USAID with people with a significant scientific background, to help make decisions on environmental health and other areas. Current funding tends to focus on biotechnology research, zoo and conservation work, and broad environmental issues; big agricultural projects are more often done by the private sector.

Daily work / Pay

Daily work includes a lot of writing; interacting with other professionals, but also with local people, to help them learn new ways of doing things; and a mix of field work and monitoring the situation once projects have been implemented.

A moderate salary is paid ($30,000-50,000), but the best things about the fellowship are the great contacts, leadership skills, knowledge of international business, and other abilities you'll pick up during your tenure. Former fellows can use their experience to continue work in the international arena, either as independent consultants or as part of a team (nonprofit agency, Governmental agency, etc). (There is little or no opportunity to stay on with USAID.)

To apply

These Fellowships are geared toward DVMS (not students) who have diverse backgrounds. International experience is a plus (e.g., with one of the organizations listed in the International jobs section, or by independent travel). The USAID fellowship requires some foreign language ability, as well as the ability to work in teams, write well (the application includes writing a "memo" or article), articulate your thoughts clearly, and take an analytical and scientific approach to problems.
AAAS, Science and Engineering Diplomacy Fellowship, 1200 New York Ave NW, Washington DC, 20005; 202 326-6600.

DEPARTMENT OF VETERANS AFFAIRS / VETERANS ADMINISTRATION (VA)

Positions in laboratory animal medicine are available for veterinarians. Most require additional degrees or board certification, but experience can be an acceptable substitute. Jobs may include organizing and directing animal research facilities; consulting and advising physicians and scientists about laboratory animals; conducting research on laboratory animals; and training medical personnel and animal technicians. A list of veterinarians who work for the Veteran's Administration is found in the AVMA *Directory*.

To apply

Some job openings for DVMs are filled via applications that were submitted through the USDA-FSIS (*see* discussion about applying for Federal jobs at the beginning of this chapter). For other positions, contact:

US Dept of Veterans Affairs, Chief Veterinary Medical Officer, 810 Vermont Ave NW Rm 15E, Washington DC 20420, 202-273-8230

ENVIRONMENTAL PROTECTION AGENCY (EPA)

Currently, the few DVMs who work for the EPA have been assigned there from the DHHS-PHS, rather than being directly employed by the EPA. (*See* DHHS-PHS, above, and Military section (PHHS Commissioned corps).

The EPA is responsible for implementing the Federal laws designed to protect human health and the environment. It conducts a variety of research, monitoring, standard-setting, and enforcement activities. As a complement to its other activities, the EPA coordinates and supports research and anti-pollution activities of state and local governments, private and public groups, individuals and educational institutions. The EPA also monitors the operations of other Federal agencies with respect to their impact on the environment. The EPA's headquarters are in Washington, D.C., with regional offices in several cities.

To apply

The EPA's *Environmental Careers Resource Guide* provides information about general career tracks within the EPA. Students can gain work experience in many environmental organizations at the local, state or Federal level, or in the private or nonprofit sectors. Several fact sheets are available, which were designed to assist environmental career speakers who are addressing students. Call or write the EPA Human Resources Office in your geographic area of interest for information about programs such as the Summer Employment Program, the Cooperative Education Program, the Federal Environmental Internship Studies Program, the EPA Management Intern Program, and the National Network for Environmental Management Studies.

Resources

Also see Environment related jobs, in International section.
US EPA Human Resources Offices, Headquarters
401 M Street, SW, Washington, DC 20460, 202-260-3267;
Job Hotline 202-260-5055
Ask for the Environmental Careers Resource Guide, and for the address and phone number of the EPA regional office nearest you.
http://www.epa.gov (click search and type jobs)

NATIONAL SCIENCE FOUNDATION (NSF)

The NSF promotes and advances scientific progress in the US by competitively awarding grants for research and education in the sciences, mathematics and engineering. The NSF hires a variety of scientists for long-term and temporary positions. There are no openings for "veterinarians" per se, but DVMS may qualify for positions such as "biologist" that require an advanced degree that could include the DVM.

To apply

NSF, 4201 Wilson Blvd. Arlington, VA 22230; 703 306-1234;
http://www.nsf.gov/
Current vacancy listings http://www.nsf.gov/oirm/
To order publications or forms 703- 306-1130, or pubs@nsf.gov
Jobline (recording) 703 306-0080 or 800 628-1487;
Human Resources Management 703 306-1182

CANADIAN ANIMAL HEALTH

Canadian Food Inspection Agency

The Canadian Federal Department of Agriculture is known as the "Canadian Food Inspection Agency" (CFIA). This department also has jurisdiction over packaging and labeling claims, and over seafood, as well as over public health inspections and all other regulatory activities to do with food. Veterinarians are hired for two basic purposes in CFIA—Animal Health and Meat Hygiene. Some may be "cross-utilized" between the two areas.

Animal Health DVMS go out to farms and investigate suspected diseases of international interest as reported by farmers and practicing veterinarians, and monitor the paperwork submitted by practice veterinarians who are certifying animals as fit for export. Their jobs involve a lot of traveling (in a Government-owned car), taking blood samples, speaking to farmers' groups, examining individual animals and herds, and doing investigative work to trace back sick animals to their original owners. Animal Health veterinarians often take blood samples from large numbers of sheep, cattle, pigs, and horses to monitor them for contagious diseases.

Meat Hygiene monitors the transportation and slaughter of animals destined to become food. Antemortem and postmortem inspections are performed. In Canada, as in the US, the veterinarian is assisted by several non-DVM inspectors who monitor every carcass and draw to the attention of the veterinarian any carcasses that are unusual.

Meat Hygiene DVMs see a lot of sick animals, which provides good experience in animal pathology. They also see the first inklings of any disease trends in farm animal populations. At some plants the DVM may work a four day week (with a longer shift each day). They are routinely required to work afternoon and midnight shifts, especially inspecting poultry.

As in the US Government, there is always a lot of paperwork; pay scales are well-defined; and advancement means managing or supervising others. Both Animal Health and Meat Hygiene positions involve some telephone time with consumers and farmers. Public relations is an important part of their function. Animal Health DVMs may travel extensively each day, especially in western Canada where farms and ranches are far apart.

Pros and cons

As with US Government jobs, the pros include good pay and benefits, regular hours, a predictable schedule, access to Federal library resources, and front-line experience in epidemiology and pathology. Cons include committee meetings, dealing with bureaucrats, the occasional adversarial relationship with meat plant management, and lack of communication between headquarters and field.

To apply

A list of addresses and phone numbers for veterinarians in a variety of positions within the Canadian Government is found in the AVMA *Directory*.

Food Production and Inspection Service, Nepean, Ontario, K1A 0Y9.
Director of Human Resources: 613-952-8000.

JOBS IN POLITICS

A variety of jobs in politics are open to veterinarians. The AVMA has four full-time veterinarians working in its Governmental Relations Division (*see* "Association jobs"). Veterinarians who have completed an AVMA Congressional Fellowship, or those with special interests in a variety of veterinary issues may be poised to work for industry or Governmental agencies as lobbyists or policy analysts. Some jobs with State Departments of Agriculture include political work. Veterinarians can also work as lobbyists for a variety of special interest groups. Lobbyists provide the Congress with information about a variety of issues. All the AVMA-GRD veterinarians are registered lobbyists, and a former State Veterinarian and Director of the Idaho State Department of Agriculture became a lobbyist for a farm bureau.

To apply / Resources

See Association jobs: AVMA-GRD
Agriculture Policy Analyst. Candace Jacobs. JAVMA 196(6) 3/15/90 pp 858-859.
Washington office staff addresses legislation affecting veterinarians. JAVMA 203(10) 11/15/93 pp 1376-1380. (About the AVMA-GRD).
AVMA *Washington Veterinary News* is published by the AVMA Governmental Relations Division. For a sample issue or subscription, contact the AVMA.

Resources: All Government jobs

Vacancy announcements

1. The US Office of Personnel Management (OPM)
Automated telephone system provides current worldwide Federal job opportunities, salary and employee benefits information, and special recruitment messages. For job information 24 hours a day, 7 days a week, call 912-757-3000. You can also record your request to have application packages, forms, and other employment-related literature mailed to you. (OPM does not automatically list vacancies from agencies with direct-hire authority). *Also see* Web site listing, that follows.

2. Federal Information Center
Call to find any Government phone numbers: 1-800-688-9889

3. Career America Connection
Federal Jobs, 24 hours a day 912-757-3000

4. Federal Career Opportunities
Federal Research Service, PO Box 1059, Vienna, VA 22183; 1-800-822-JOBS or 703-281-0200. A biweekly publication listing thousands of currently available Federal jobs, nationwide and overseas positions organized by job series within each agency, contact names and phone numbers for application information, vacancy numbers, and brief job descriptions. Each issue contains helpful articles on the Federal hiring process. (Note: this information is available free from various Government sources, but you might find it easier to read in this organized publication.)

5. Federal Information Exchange (FEDIX)
Provides electronic access to Federal research and education opportunities: research opportunities, equipment grants, program contacts, education scholarships and grants, current events, and minority opportunities. Sponsored by the DOE, DOC, DOA, FAA, NASA, and several other agencies. http://www.fie.com/

Groups

1. See the current AVMA *Directory* for current and updated addresses of many of the groups or associations listed throughout this book. It also has lists of Officials in charge of animal disease control; State Public Health Veterinarians of the US; Officials in charge of state meat inspection; and USDA and US Dept of Health and Human Services offices. AVMA, 1931 N Meacham Rd, Suite 100, Schaumburg IL 60173-4360, 800-248-2862

2. American Association of Public Health Veterinarians
c/o Dr. David Sasaki, Dept of Health, Epidemiology; Rm 107, PO Box 3378, Honolulu HI 96801

3. US Public Health Service Veterinarians
Dr. Michael Blackwell, Metro Park North 2, Rm 4-84, FDA Ctr for Veterinary Medicine, Rockville MD 20855, 301-594-1798

4. *National Association of Federal Veterinarians*
Has a helpful information sheet, "Sources of Federal employment opportunities for veterinarians." Dr. Boyle, 1101 Vermont St NW, Suite 710, Washington DC 20005-3521, 202-289-6334 (or see AVMA *Directory* for current address).
5. *Federal Research Service.* A private group specializing in helping people get Government jobs; has lots of resources, including a newsletter, "Federal Career Opportunities," with an extensive, up-to-date listing of job openings and tips about the job application process. 243 Church Street NW, Suite 200W; PO Box 1059; Vienna VA 22183-1059 http://www.fedjobs.com info@fedjobs.com 800-822-5027 or 703-281-0200 Fax: 703-281-7639

Online resources

To get an immediate, current list of all Federal job openings and a job application, get online and check out some Web sites.
1. *OPM: US Office of Personnel Management*
Find an online application at their Web site
http://www.usajobs.opm.gov/
Or, dial 912-757-3100 with your modem for job information from their electronic bulletin board. You can also reach the board through the Internet at host FJOB.MAIL.OPM.GOV. After looking at the OPM's Web site, you'll see that the variety of Federal jobs for which you qualify is vastly broader than you'd ever imagined. Scroll through the entire list of job openings rather than going straight to words you think of first ("veterinarian"). (For example, a recent search revealed a listing for a good-paying job as a "technical information specialist" with the National Cancer Institute, that had requirements many DVMs would meet). There are specific instructions for applying for each job on the Web sites where they are listed.
2. *Applying for a Federal Job*
http://helix.nih.gov:8001/jobs/of510.html
3. *File Resource Library*
Federal Job Openings listed by the Office of Personnel Management
http://hi-tec.twc.state.tx.us/fedjobs.htm
4. *Federal Jobs Application Forms Editor for Windows*
Turns blank paper into a completed OF-612's, SF-171's, OF-306's on your PC. http://www.cybercomm.net/~digibook/formedit.html
5. *Computerized Form 171 Advanced!*
Prints the Standard Form 171 on plain paper.
http://www.netis.com/appolo/cf171.htm
6. *FedWorld Information Network*
703-487-4219   http://www.fedworld.gov

Government Web sites

1. USDA vacancy announcements http://www.usda.gov/da/employ.html
2. USDA Human resources division
http://www.reeusda.gov/new/hrd/hrdmob.html

3. USDA Research, Education and Economics Home Page
http://www.reeusda.gov/ree/
4. CSREES Cooperative State Research Education and Extension Service
http://www.reeusda.gov/
5. CSREES job opportunities
http://www.reeusda.gov/new/hrd/novlist3.htm
6. APHIS http://www.aphis.usda.gov/
7. APHIS vacancy announcements
http://www.aphis.usda.gov/mb/mrphr/vacancy.html
8. APHIS Veterinary Services http://www.aphis.usda.gov/vs/
9. APHIS, VS, CEAH, E-mail: nahms_web@aphis.usda.gov
10. APHIS Veterinary Biologics http://aphisweb.aphis.usda.gov/bbep/vb/
11. NIH National Institutes of Health
http://www.aamc.org/research/adhocgp/aboutnih.htm
12. PHHS Public Health Svc Commissioned Corps
http://phs.os.dhhs.gov/phs/corps/welcom1.html
13. CDC Center for Disease Control and Prevention http://www.cdc.gov/
14. CEAH Centers for Epidemiology and Animal Health
http://www.aphis.usda/gov/vs/ceah/
15. FDA Food and Drug Administration http://www.fda.gov/
16. FDA Center for Veterinary Medicine http://www.cvm.fda.gov/
17. FSIS Food Safety and Inspection Service http://www.usda.gov/fsis/
18. EPA Environmental Protection Agency http://www.epa.gov/epahome/
19. FWS Fish and Wildlife Service http://www.fws.gov/
20. NSF National Science Foundation http://www.nsf.gov/
21. To find more, use a Web search tool and enter the name of the
organization you want.

Books

1. *The Book of US Government Jobs: Where They Are, What's Available,
and How to Get One.* Includes extensive list of resources, addresses, etc.
Dennis V. Damp, 1996.
2. *Applying For Federal Jobs: A Guide to Writing Successful Applications
and Resumes for the Job You Want in Government* Patricia B. Wood,
1995.
3. *The Entrepreneur's Guide to Doing Business With the Federal
Government.* How to sell your products or services to the Government. C
Bevers, L Christie, L Price. Prentice Hall 1989.
4. *Federal Job Winner's Tips series* Federal Research Service, Inc., PO
Box 1059, Vienna, VA 22183-1059; 1-800-822-JOBS or 703-281-0200
(Not a Government organization). A series of five booklets to guide you
through the Federal hiring process to career success. (How to Start Your
Job Search; How to Select Your Occupation; How to Prepare Your
Application; How to Interview for Job Openings; and How to Change
Careers Within Government).
5. *The Government Job Finder.* Daniel Lauber. Directory to over 1,000 job
sources, including periodicals with ads on Government jobs; job
hotlines; and job matching services.

6. *The Directory of Federal Jobs and Employers.* Ron and Caryl Krannich. Contact information on hundreds of Federal Government agencies; includes names, addresses, and phone numbers of personnel offices and job hotlines; and describes the work of specific agencies. 1996.

7. *The Complete Guide to Public Employment.* Ron and Caryl Krannich. A guide to public-oriented careers. How to find jobs with Federal, state, and local governments; associations; contractors; foundations; and research and political groups. 1995.

Articles

1. *Professional profile: Crusading for unconventional careers.* Susan Kahler. Profile of Dr. Michael J. Blackwell, chief veterinary officer for the US Public Health Service and Deputy Director of the FDA-CVM. JAVMA 208(3) 2/1/96 pp 332-333.

2. *And why epidemiology?* H. Michael Maetz. JAVMA 190(8) 4/15/87 pp 970-972.

3. *US Public Health Service training and career development opportunities for veterinarians.* Robert Whitney. (Exact descriptions are outdated because of Government reorganization). JAVMA 193(4) 8/15/88 pp 422-427.

4. *Sources of Federal employment opportunities for veterinarians.* Edward Menning. (exact descriptions are outdated because of Government reorganization). JAVMA 193(6) 9/15/88 pp 658-661.

5. *Federal Service.* Alwynelle Ahl. JAVMA 193(12) 12/15/88 pp 1486-1487.

6. *The Congressional Science Fellowship.* Martha Gearhart. JAVMA 196 (5) 3/1/90 pp 721-724.

7. *Agricultural policy analyst.* Candace Jacobs. JAVMA 196(6) 3/15/90 pp 858-859.

CHAPTER 17

THE UNIFORMED SERVICES

About 500 veterinarians currently work in the uniformed services (which includes the military and the Public Health Service Commissioned Corps). These jobs can be in any state or overseas, but are concentrated in Maryland, Texas, and US Possessions (e.g., Puerto Rico, Guam). A higher percentage of graduates of Auburn, Colorado State, Kansas State, Oklahoma State, and Texas A & M are working in the military than are graduates of other veterinary schools.

Below are descriptions of a variety of military positions. Since the specifics may change over time, be sure to get current information from your military recruiter. Better yet, attend meetings where military DVMs are present (e.g., the AVMA annual meeting) and ask them about how they like their jobs. A cautionary note from many people within the Army: "Be very careful of Recruiters! They will tell you exactly what you *want* to hear!" I found that to be somewhat true, in that recruiters were vague and overly optimistic in telling me how much control military DVMs have over where they are stationed, compared with what military DVMs actually reported.

If you don't mind the lack of control over where you live and how often you move, the uniformed services are a great way to gain experience for future jobs and to get any further education paid for.

The Navy and Coast Guard don't directly hire veterinary officers. Veterinarians may be assigned to these facilities as part of the PHS commissioned corps (see below).

AIR FORCE

Veterinarians may apply to the Air Force as Public Health Officers (PHOS) in the Biomedical Sciences Corps. Their field of work, public health, focuses on disease control. Air Force DVMS work in the area of human public health. They do not work on animals at all (Army DVMS work on any Air Force animals that need veterinary attention). Air Force public health work can be a good stepping-stone to non-military jobs with state Departments of Health (*see* State Jobs).

Daily work

PHOS work on disease surveillance, zoonoses control, food inspection, and food facility sanitation. They basically help operate a public health department for their base. That work can involve sexually transmitted diseases, deployment medicine, immunizations, occupational medicine (ergonomics, hearing and respiratory protection), or vector surveillance and control.

PHOS work with environmental and disease hazards during disasters and wartime situations. They may collect and analyze data from foreign countries and advise the military of potential health threats. The PHO is in a supervisory position with a staff that assists in these endeavors. PHOS may work with other health professionals in the areas of preventive medicine and epidemiology.

Communicable disease control includes gathering and analyzing epidemiologic data, and assisting physicians in determining treatment and disease control. PHOS may gather information on medical factors that may affect the capability of military forces when they deploy, and recommending preventive measures. PHOS inspect dining facilities for proper food service standards.

Initial assignments are for three years. When you are recruited for an Air Force position, you can make a specific request to be stationed in one place. You are guaranteed to be placed there, but there's no guarantee you won't be moved at any time. From there, you can go to a variety of locations, based on your application or the AF's needs. In general, you are moved about every three years. Although you can request a change in location, the needs of the AF comes first. There are at most three PHOS at one facility. You cannot usually get overseas assignments (including AK and HI) on you first assignment.

The Air Force offers deployment "opportunities" (you're "selected," you don't choose). PHOS are part of a preventive medicine team that goes into countries ahead of air crew flight lines to set up preventive medical and food safety programs for the troops. These assignments usually last no more than 90 days, and can be as short as 2-3 weeks.

Pay

Air Force PHO DVMS enter active duty as Captains (unless they entered veterinary school after three years of undergraduate work, and don't have a BS, in which case they start as First Lieutenants). After an initial course at the School of Aerospace Medicine in Texas (12 weeks of training focusing on public health; four weeks of basic military training), they are sent to their assignments.

After their first three years in the Air Force (first appointment) PHOS are strongly encouraged to get an MPH or another degree. The Air Force offers two ways to do so: either continue in your job and pursue the degree part-time (the AF pays 75% of tuition costs), or attend school full time on a full AF scholarship—with some flexibility in where you attend school (they'll tell you that you can apply anywhere you want, but they "assist" you with that selection and have final say in where you go). With either route you are obligated to "repay" your schooling with several years of work in the Air Force. With your additional education, you may go into teaching, research, or a commander position in a hospital or clinic.

To apply/Resources

1-800-423-USAF. Chief, Military Public Health, HQ USAF SGPA, Bolling AFB, DC 20332-5113, 202-767-1838 (Note: you may have to contact more than one recruiter; an Air Force medical recruiter incorrectly told

me that the Air Force did not hire any DVMs. He was unaware that DVMs are hired as part of the Biomedical Sciences Corps.)
http://www.airforce.com/visitor/carrctr/medical/medical.html
http://www.airforce.com
Biomedical Sciences Corps (Air Force). Deneice Jackson. JAVMA 197(10) 11/15/90pp1313-1314.
Air Force environmental health services. J. Kevin Grayson. JAVMA 192(2) 1/15/88pp169-170.

ARMY

The US Army Veterinary Corps hires veterinarians to care for pets and horses; for food inspection; for disaster relief; and to conduct biomedical research (after they help you get an advanced degree). All DVMs enter the Army Veterinary Corps with at least the rank of Captain. To qualify, you must be under 33 years old (too old? *See* "Public Health Service Commissioned Corps," below).

The Army Veterinary Corps conducts and oversees all Department of Defense veterinary missions at over 1,000 locations in more than 40 countries. DVMs serve in three areas: research and development, food safety, and animal medicine. They are responsible for disease control, biomedical research and development, epidemiology or public health, and management.

Daily work

After military orientation and food inspection/public health courses (each lasting several months), Army DVMs are assigned to work at a military base. They are responsible for inspection of all meat that comes into the commissaries (military grocery stores). They perform basic medical procedures on the pets of military active duty and family members (who choose to use that facility). They also give medical and surgical care to Government-owned animals, including laboratory animals, military working dogs, marine mammals or ceremonial horses. The Army is responsible for providing care to all working dogs and other animals for all the Departments of Defense—the Air Force, Navy, and Army. Only preventive medicine is done. The amount of time spent working in the base veterinary clinic versus doing meat inspection will vary with the location's needs.

Human disease cases suspected to be of animal origin may require quarantines and epidemiologic investigations. The Army DVM's duties may include public health education programs, stray animal control, and liaison with local disease control authorities, or monitoring programs, which identify the existence of zoonotic diseases in wild animals. Veterinarians may also initiate and supervise pet-facilitated therapy programs. These programs include small animal screening for hospital visitation and therapeutic horsemanship.

The Army's mission requires operation in a field environment. In the event of a national emergency, the veterinarian helps protect the livestock industry, providing foreign countries with assistance in animal disease control and in providing emergency medical support in veterinary-related areas. The Veterinary Corps also trains officers to provide support in areas of Low Intensity Conflict. Special emphasis has been placed on training for deployment to areas of Central and South America and Asia.

Veterinarians are also involved in food safety. They provide scientific checks during procurement, storage, transportation, and distribution of food products. (For details about the daily work of meat inspection, *see* the Federal Civilian Jobs section: USDA-FSIS.)

Army veterinarians develop vaccines and antidotes to protect troops from the possible effects of biological and chemical warfare. They also study food and animal contamination that can result from it. Almost a third of all veterinary officers are engaged in biomedical and subsistence research and development for the military. Before entering biomedical research, or following initial assignments, DVMS are offered an advanced training residency in laboratory animal medicine or pathology at one of several Army institutes.

Army DVMS might work in other agencies of the Department of Defense—the overseas Navy medical research units, the Armed Forces Radiobiology Research Institute, the Armed Forces Institute of Pathology, the US Army Medical Research and Development Command, or in many Department of Defense clinical investigation activities in the US and overseas. They also may be assigned to an Air Force or Navy research laboratory.

Pros and cons

Being in the Army means being flexible about moving to differ-ent areas of the country or the world. You can have fun with this, learning about and enjoying different cultures and in-terests. You can also suffer, being placed in an area you don't enjoy, or moving more often than you'd like. According to one source, relocation is expected every 24-36 months. When moving to new assignments, payment of travel expenses and shipping charges for families and personal goods is provided. You can request assignment to a certain country, but aren't guaranteed placement there. Daily travel depends on your duty position; with that comes a per diem payment. Those DVMs with a non-military spouse are likely to have trouble because of the frequent moves and, sometimes, the travel requirements (daily or weekly travel).

The clinical medicine you'll practice is basic preventive medicine; if you want to do a lot of procedures and see a variety of cases, you most likely won't find that. In most cases, there are no emergency calls. You'll have limited animal work, endless paperwork, and potential for long-term deployments.

For example, one position would be as an *officer in charge of a Veterinary Services squad*, responsible for preparing sol-diers (technicians and food inspectors) to deploy anywhere in the world in support of US forces. Soldiers are prepared to move into the field and to establish and operate a food in-spection and animal medicine program within 72 hours. Their primary mission is food inspection with a secondary mission as first line care for military working dogs.

Long-term overseas positions are also available. A year's assignment in the US is required before being sent overseas. On assignment in other countries, duties can include inspec-tion of foods and commercial food establishments, public health support, herd health, and food animal medicine. Higher-ranking officers or those who have completed further training may become instructors or supervisors of these pro-grams. For example, one position would involve traveling around Europe as an inspector of dairy processing plants that sell dairy products to the military.

Pay and benefits

Salaries and benefits are good. Advancement in rank is competitive and based on a time scale. Pay increases are based on a published schedule. Retirement is available after 20 years with 30% of pay and continued health benefits.

Benefits include a 30-day paid annual vacation; all Federal holidays off; regular hours (most of the time); convenient post exchanges and commissaries; medical benefits for you and your dependents; tax-free housing allowance, or Government housing provided in some military communities; tax-free subsistence (food) allowance; a low-cost term life insurance policy; a non-contributory retirement program; and disability retirement pay. Women report that costs of pregnancy and quality of child care are excellent. You may have access to officers' clubs, tennis courts, golf courses, swimming pools, libraries, theaters, hobby and craft shops, and other complimentary services.

All Army Officers must complete a series of educational courses in their branch as well as in the management and command structures of the military as a whole. All medical branches (veterinarians, physicians, and dentists) spend several weeks in Fort Sam Houston, Texas. After that, all Veterinary Corps (vcs) take a 3-month course in Chicago (mainly learning food inspection).

To qualify for positions and promotions, vc Officers take courses such as the "Officers Advanced Course" for AMEDS (Army Medical) Officers. To be promoted to Lieutenant Colonel, they take the "Command and General Staff Course." If they join a Civil Affairs Unit, they take additional courses in civil affairs taught at the JFK special warfare school Ft. Bragg, NC. They can also take a number of courses from the US Navy Correspondence course center in Florida on subjects of personal interest such as marine navigation and shiphandling. The Army encourages board certification for continued promotion.

Army DVMs also have access to continuing education, including the pursuit of additional degrees. (However, training opportunities are limited to those that the military needs at that time.) There are long-term civilian training opportunities in public health, lab animal medicine, pathology, and a few clinical specialty slots with full pay and benefits. Army DVMs can compete for specialized education in civilian institutions leading to graduate degrees in public health, laboratory animal medicine, veterinary microbiology, pathology, physiology, toxicology, pharmacology, and food technology, for example. Army preceptorship programs are also available in veterinary pathology and laboratory animal medicine.

To apply/Resources

Contact any regional army *medical* recruiter, or:

USA PERSCOM, TAPC-OPH-VC, 200 Stovall St, Alexandria VA 22332-0417; 703-325-2360; 1-800-USA-ARMY or 703-325-2360 (ok to call collect).
http://vetpath1.afip.mil/Vet_Services/vs.html   http://www.goarmy.com   http://vetpath1.afip.mil/vetcorps/vc_1.html
US Army Veterinary Corps; Chief, US Army Veterinary Corps, Attn: MCVS; 2050 Worth Rd, Ft Sam Houston TX 78234-6000, 210-221-6522
Diverse opportunities in the army veterinary corps. Frederick Angulo. JAVMA 190(4) 2/15/87pp366-367.

US PUBLIC HEALTH SERVICE (USPHS) COMMISSIONED CORPS

The Commissioned Corps is an all-officer organization that provides employment opportunities for health professionals and students. As part of the Department of Health and Human Services (DHHS), the Commissioned Corps has officers assigned to all of the Public Health Services Agencies and Program offices (*See* "Civilian Federal Jobs" for details about these agencies.)

USPHS officers are most likely to be assigned to the CDC, EPA, FDA, or NIH. In addition, commissioned officers are also assigned to certain agencies outside the PHS, to help meet their health professional staffing needs. At the professional level, each of the PHS Agencies and Program Offices, and those non-DHHS Agencies that use officers, determines those positions best suited for a commissioned officer and seeks the most qualified candidates.

Individuals are commissioned in the corps for a career with the PHS rather than for a position in a particular program area. The assignment should provide experience and/or training that will prepare the officer for possible future assignments. The Corps benefits are similar to those provided to officers in the other Uniformed Services. Most positions that would be open to a veterinarian are in biomedical animal research or epidemiology. Typical positions include laboratory animal veterinarian, veterinary pathologist, epidemiologist, and regulatory veterinarian. The Corps DVM is assisted in taking an active role in finding a desired position.

Sample PHS Jobs

Regulatory Veterinarian: Reviews and evaluates applications of new animal drugs, devices, food, food additives and other chemicals intended for use in animals. Considers adequate labeling, the effects of various agents on animal systems, and questions of drug safety or effectiveness. Determines the need for revised labeling or withdrawal of a drug from the market. Informs the application sponsors of any deficiencies in their applications. Helps to plan and implement various disease studies. Can advance to supervisory positions that include more authority and autonomy, including serving as an expert Federal consultant to industry on drug approval policy. Lower level jobs require only a DVM; promotion requires more experience, and advancement to the highest level may require board certification or another advanced degree.

Staff Epidemiologist or Pathologist: These positions require an additional degree or residency. Note, however, that you must only have completed the coursework for an additional degree—you needn't have been awarded the degree itself.

Pay

The Commissioned Corps offers a base salary; medical and dental coverage; low-cost life insurance; 30 days paid vacation each year; a non-contributory retirement plan; and travel, housing and subsistence allowances.

The Corps is a great way to get an overview of potential Government jobs. You can use this experience to move into a civilian Federal job, or you can remain in the Corps for a long-term career. Many of the jobs you could get via the Corps are the same as those you could get as a civilian, so it's important to weigh the pros and cons of being a uniformed versus a civilian employee. The Corps may offer a higher or a lower salary for the same type of work, depending on the specific position. Ask the PHS for a copy of their informative paper, "Comparison of Civil Service and Commissioned Corps."

To apply

To be appointed, you must be under 44 years old and be willing to be assigned wherever needed (although you are encouraged to get involved in the search for an appropriate position). All initial appointments are made to the Reserve Corps, and reserve officers serve a 3-year probationary period. Advanced training is encouraged for professionals while they are in the Corps.

US Public Health Service Commissioned Corps Recruitment, 5600 Fishers Lane Room 4A-07, Rockville MD 20857-0001 or

USPHS Chief Veterinary Officer, 7500 Standish Place, Rockville MD 20855; 1-800-279-1605; 1-800-279-1606; recruit@psc.ssw.dhhs.gov

Job announcements http://phs.os.dhs.gov/psc/hrs/dhhsjobs.txt

Resources

Links to related sites http://phs.os.dhhs.gov/phs/phs.html
General information http://phs.os.dhhs.gov/phs/corps/welcom1.html
For a brochure, "Public Health Service Commissioned Corps," request CCPM Pamphlet No. 66 from The Dept of Health & Human Services, Program Support Center, Human Resources Service, Division of Commissioned Personnel, 5600 Fishers Lane Room 4A-07, Rockville MD 20857-0001.

US Public Health Service Veterinarians
Dr. Michael Blackwell, Metro Park North 2, Rm 4-84, FDA Ctr for Veterinary Medicine, Rockville MD 20855, 301-594-1798

PHS *veterinarians help islanders weather storm's aftermath.* JAVMA 208(1) 1/1/96 pp 15.

US Public Health Service training and career development opportunities for veterinarians. Robert Whitney. (Exact descriptions are outdated because of Government reorganization.) JAVMA 193(4) 8/15/88 pp 422-427.

PART-TIME WORK IN THE UNIFORMED SERVICES

Not all military jobs require a full-time commitment. For part-time duty and supplemental income of several thousand dollars per year, contact:

USA Reserve   Attn: ARPC-OPS-MC   Cdr, ARPERCEN 9700 Page Blvd, St Louis MO 63132-5200, 314-538-2121; 800-325-4973

Openings that are currently available can be obtained from:

HQ, VETCOM, Ft Sam Houston TX 78234; 210-221-6522.

Air National Guard; NGB/DPR; Andrews AFB, MD 20331; 301-981-8569

Air Force Reserve: 1800-257-1212

National Guard, AMEDD Procurement, Army National Guard Readiness Center, Attn: NGB-ARP-HN; 111 S George Mason Dr, Arlington VA 22204-1382, 703-607-7145

FUTURE GOALS FOR THE PROFESSION

The fact that there is a need for this book points to a void within the veterinary profession. Will we rise to meet the challenge of molding the future of veterinary medicine? Although many DVMS voice concern about low pay and lack of job opportunties, their concerns are diverted by long discussions of whether or not a problem exists.

I submit that if enough veterinarians perceive a problem, then one does exist. Let's focus our attention, then, on finding solutions. While I worked on gathering information for this book, I became aware of one big obstacle to the "broadening" of the veterinary profession beyond private practice—a lack of easy access to good information about the variety of career choices available to DVMS.

All the organizations, agencies, and groups listed in this book can help by:

• Establishing externships for students *and for veterinarians* to learn about careers with their organizations.
• Re-examining their job descriptions and considering the wide array of positions that DVMS may fill.
• Contacting the AVMA's Placement Service whenever a job opening occurs.
• Analyzing why certain schools have a higher percentage of graduates entering government or industry, and helping other schools create similar programs.

• Creating written job descriptions that are easily obtained by those who contact their human resources or personnel departments.

The AVMA can serve as a model and can lead the way by:

• Creating clear written job descriptions of positions within its own organization, and encouraging industry and other organizations to do the same.
• Publicizing the salaries it pays its DVM employees, and encouraging industry and other organizations to do the same.
• Focusing AVMA Foundation money or other available resources on distance learning (e.g., via computer), or short courses for DVMs that focus on skills needed to obtain non-practice jobs, or that give an overview of various non-practice jobs. (The Foundation does sponsor student precepteeships in informatics, epidemiology, and laboratory animal medicine.)

Our veterinary teaching hospitals can help by:

• Revising the pre-veterinary requirements to reflect more business and public health.
• Exposing students to their choices as early as possible, rather than giving them a cursury overview as seniors.
• Establishing short courses for DVMs that focus on skills needed to obtain non-practice jobs, or that give an overview of various non-practice jobs.
• Providing students with more details about non-practice career paths, by
   • hosting guest speakers who work in those jobs
   • providing courses in epidemiology and public health
   • assisting students in finding externships outside of private practice

Both our teaching hospitals and the AVMA can help by:

• Analyzing the patterns of job change among veterinarians—specifically asking:
   • What percentage of DVMs end up in jobs different than the ones on which they'd planned?

- On average, how many years passed before they made the change?
- How can the AVMA and the teaching hospitals use this information to help DVMs who are approaching this transitional period?

One problem is that schools must prepare the future DVM for passing the National Board Examination. The NBE, in turn, is meant to protect the public from harm, and thus focuses on traditional veterinary practice. With this criteria as the main focus of our teaching hospitals, we will always have a problem in "diverting" new graduates to non-practice careers.

A good part of the discussion for change in veterinary teaching hospitals has been about whether students should be allowed to choose a "track" and limit their studies to one species. One concern is that a student who, for instance, tracks in equine medicine, cannot easily change to small animal medicine in the future. Lost in this discussion is the realization that *schools already track students*—in private practice. Few or none of today's students are easily able to change to non-practice career paths. Will designated licensure or limited training (to certain species) during veterinary school give us the results we need, or will it only serve to further limit the choices that DVMs have when or if they want to change career paths in the future?

Our challenge as a profession is in protecting the public while still planning for the future of veterinary medicine. All veterinarians must ask themselves what they can do to effect change.

RESOURCES

This section is essential reading. If you are serious about researching job possibilities, approach your search as a job in itself, or as a class that you are taking. Read everything you can get your hands on. I've listed sources of further information in two ways: general references, here, and specific references, in each section. *See the introduction to find out how to obtain these materials.*

The American Veterinary Medical Association's
MEMBERSHIP DIRECTORY AND RESOURCE MANUAL
This reference is an essential resource for everyone. Take a few hours to closely look at what's in the *AVMA Directory*, if you haven't done so before. It lists many of the organizations, schools, and people you will want to contact to get further information about certain jobs. Most veterinarians are members of the AVMA, and thus get the directory mailed to them every year. If you don't have a copy, you can order one from the AVMA, or borrow one from another veterinarian or from a veterinary school library. Also check the AVMA web site, since this information may someday be available online.
AVMA, 1931 N Meacham Rd #100, Schaumburg IL 60173; 1-800-248-2862; http://www.avma.org

AVMA CAREER PLACEMENT SERVICE Matches job applicants with job openings. Provides career counseling.
AVMA Career Development Center. 1931 N Meacham Rd #100
Schaumburg IL 60173. 1-800-248-2862 (Also see AVMA web site)

Organizations
1. *AgriCareers job placement service*
(712) 779-3300 fax (712) 779-3366
Hwy. 92 West Massena, Iowa 50853
(515) 394-3148 fax (515) 394-3406
Hwy 63 South New Hampton, Iowa 50659
http://www.netins.net/showcase/jmaas/agricareers/
2. *The Association of Part-Time Professionals*
PO Box 3419, Alexandria, VA 22302

Veterinary Web sites and online information
1. AVMA web site has job listings. http://www.avma.org
NOAH, The *Network of Animal Health,* is sponsored by the AVMA.
http://www.avma.org/network.html
2. NetVet (links to a wide variety of veterinary pages for veterinarians
and pet owners; list of listservs)   http://www.avma.org/netvet/
3. America Online is the host for VIN, The *Veterinary Information
Network.* VIN, 1411 West Covell Blvd, Suite 106-131, Davis CA 95616;
800 700-4636;   http://www.vetinfonet.com/
4. VetNet (for veterinarians only) http://www.vet.net
5. List of VetMed/Animal Conferences
http://duke.usask.ca/~ladd/vconfram.htm
6. Veterinary Medicine Libraries
http://duke.usask.ca/~ladd/vet_libraries.html
7. VETS - CAB Abstracts: Veterinary Science & Medicine
http://www.rs.ch/www/rs/ds/VETS.HTML

Web sites for job hunting
Most company and government Web sites have information
about job opportunities. You will find more Web sites, specific to each job, listed in the appropriate chapters.

Finding a specific organization: Since there are new Web
sites being built each day, the best thing to do is to learn how
to *search for what you want.* "Search engines" are Web sites
that you go to, that help you search for other Web sites.

Good search engines
Alta Vista http://www.altavista.digital.com/
Yahoo! http://www.yahoo.com/
Excite http://www.excite.com

Job listings

(Also see the AVMA web site, listed previously)

1. OPM: US Office of Personnel Management—Federal Jobs
http://www.usajobs.opm.gov/
2. Veterinary Career Resources   http://netvet.wustl.edu/vcareer.htm
3. Job Bank http://www.ajb.dni.us
4. Veterinary Jobs http://www.showcom.com/user/vetjobs.htm
5. AgriCareers (job placement service)
http://www.netins.net/showcase/jmaas/agricareers/
6. The Career Superstore http://www.impactpublications.com/gov.html
7. Small Business Administration   http://www.sba.gov/
8. Other job sites:
http://www.careermosaic.com
http://www.careerpath.com
http://www.espan.com
http://www.Career-path.com
http://www.jobcenter.com
http://www.cweb.com
http://www.classifieds.yahoo.com
http://www.monster.com

Electronic mailing lists

These are informal "discussion groups" that cater to specific interests.
New lists are constantly formed, and old ones disbanded; see the NetVet
Web site (above) for a current list of veterinary-related lists (varies from
beef cattle veterinarians to veterinary informatics groups).

Vetplus electronic mail list—for veterinary professionals. See this Web
site for information. http://pserv.vet.cornell.edu/~vetplus

Books

General career and life books

1. *70 Suggestions for a Shorter, Smarter Job Hunt.* Am Soc of Association
Executives, 1996 (202-626-ASAE; fax 371-8825)
2. *Executive Job-changing Workbook.* John Lucht. Am Soc of Association
Executives 1994.
3. *Future Directions For Veterinary Medicine.* Pew National Veterinary
Education Program. The Pew Charitable Trust, 1989.
4. *The Lifetime Career Manager: New strategies for a new era.* James
Cabrera. Am Soc of Association Executives, 1995.
5. *Make Yourself Memorable.* S Sherman & V Sherman. Am Soc of
Association Executives, 1996.
6. *Planning Your Veterinary Career.* American Animal Hospital
Association, 1987. PO Box 150899, Denver CO 80215
7. *Rites of Passage at $100,000+:* The insider's guide to absolutely
everything about executive job-changing. John Lucht. Am Soc of
Association Executives 1993.

8. *Robert Gerberg's Job Changing System.* R. Gerberg 1970, 1984.
Specific advice about pursuing a job change.
9. *The Three Boxes of Life—and how to get out of them.* Richard N. Bolles,
1978 (old but definitely *not* outdated!) Essential reading for anyone
feeling "burned out."
10. *Veterinary demographic annual reports* Gives breakdown by state and
type of employment (gov't, industry, etc). Obtain from the AVMA 1931 N
Meacham Rd, Suite 100, Schaumburg IL 60173-4360; 800-248-2862
11. *Veterinary Medicine in Economic Transition.* Malcolm Getz, 1997.
12. *What Color is Your Parachute?* Richard Bolles. The classic job-
changing guide.
13. *Your Money or Your Life.* Joe Dominguez & Vicki Robin. Essential
reading for those who feel they cannot make a change because they
can't afford it. (Tells you *how* to do it!)
14. *What Next? Career Strategies after 35.* Jack Falvey, 1978. A good pep
talk for those feeling "stuck," uncertain, or afraid to make a change.
15. *The 1995 AAHA Report.* American Animal Hospital Association. A
study of the companion animal services market.

Books: Part-time/temporary work

1. *Part Time Professional* by Diane S. Rothberg & Barbara Ensor Cook
Acropolis Books, Ltd, Washington DC; 1985
2. *The Temp Worker's Handbook* W Lewis & N Schuman
Amacom:American Management Association; 1988

Articles

1. *A horse of another color: The accounting bug bit.* Marsha Heinke, DVM
CPA. Veterinary Forum 8/93 pp60.
2. *Changes in the number and geographic distribution of US veterinarians
employed by public or corporate organizations, 1980-1990 and 1990-
1995.* Brad Gehrke. JAVMA 209(8) 10/15/96 pp1404-1405.
3. *The Classics: the complete guide to the best business and management
books ever written.* Jim Collins. Inc 12/96 pp53-65
4. *Dual degrees equip veterinarians for novel careers.* (Counseling, law,
business, cultural anthropology, human medicine, dentist.) Paul Zuziak.
JAVMA 197(4) 8/15/90 pp443-448.
5. *Get more from your benefits package* (for part-time DVMs). Working
Woman, 10/94 pp23-25.
6. *The new job squeeze: Women pushed into part-time work.* Karen Judd.
Ms. magazine, May/June 1994 pp86-90 (discusses problems with part-
time work; good reading for both men and women.)
7. *Professional profile: Crusading for unconventional careers.* Susan
Kahler. JAVMA, 208(3) 2/1/96 pp 332-333. US Public Health Service
Veterinarian (FDA).
8. *Stagnant wages, increasing debt burden: Profession needs a plan.*
Kenneth Bovee. DVM Newsmagazine, 29 (3) 3/97 pp 1 et seq

JAVMA series

The JAVMA published a series of articles called "Career Pathways in Veterinary Medicine" several years ago. Although some of the specific information is outdated, these make great reading to get a general idea of what's involved in certain jobs.

1. Laboratory animal medicine: no typical workday. Lynn Anderson. JAVMA 189(11) 12/1/86 pp 1425-1427.

2. Swine consultation practice: A telephone and a computer modem. Gregg BeVier. JAVMA 190(2) 1/15/87 pp 154-156.

3. Diverse opportunities in the army veterinary corps. Frederick Angulo. JAVMA 190(4) 2/15/87 pp 366-367.

4. And why epidemiology? H. Michael Maetz. JAVMA 190(8) 4/15/87 pp 970-972.

5. Consultant to the food animal industry. Lawrence Price. JAVMA 190(10) 5/15/87 pp 1274-1276.

6. Directing a veterinary technician program. Karen Hrapkiewicz. JAVMA 190(12) 6/15/87 pp 1538-1539.

7. Careers in academia: Teaching and research in the basic sciences. Bradford Smith. JAVMA 191(2) 7/15/87 pp 188-190.

8. Animal care and control center. Dan Parmer. JAVMA 191(6) 9/15/87 pp 658-659.

9. Poultry veterinary medicine. John Donahoe. JAVMA 191(12) 12/15/87 pp 1530-1531.

10. Air Force environmental health services. J. Kevin Grayson. JAVMA 192(2) 1/15/88 pp 169-170.

11. The last thing this country needs is another attorney. Thomas Allison. JAVMA 193(2) 7/15/88 pp 181-183.

12. US Public Health Service training and career development opportunities for veterinarians. Robert Whitney. JAVMA 193(4) 8/15/88 pp 422-427.

13. Sources of Federal employment opportunities for veterinarians. Edward Menning. JAVMA 193(6) 9/15/88 pp 658-661.

14. Veterinary clinical nutrition. Rebecca Remillard. JAVMA 193(10) 11/15/88 pp 1238-1240.

15. Federal service. Alwynelle Ahl. JAVMA 193(12) 12/15/88 pp 1486-1487.

16. Industrial medicine in the land of Oz. Elizabeth Hodgkins. JAVMA 195(7) 10/1/89 pp 922-923 (Pet food co. work).

17. The congressional science fellowship. Martha Gearhart. JAVMA 196 (5) 3/1/90 pp 721-724.

18. Agricultural policy analyst. Candace Jacobs. JAVMA 196(6) 3/15/90 pp 858-859.

19. Back to school again: First step toward a new career. Gary Jones. JAVMA 196(8) 4/15/90 pp1236-1237. (Dairy practitioner does clinical microbiology research, leading to grad studies in molecular biology).

20. Biomedical sciences corps (air force). Deneice Jackson. JAVMA 197(10) 11/15/90 pp1313-1314.

21. *Industrial veterinary medicine: Career in a young company.* David Schabdach. JAVMA 197(12) 12/15/90 pp1592-1594.

22. *A veterinarian's role in aquaculture.* John Pitts. JAVMA 198(2) 1/15/91 pp 234-236.

23. *Large-scale swine production.* Michael Terrill. JAVMA 198(4) 2/15/91 pp 563-565.

24. *State animal health organizations.* Dennis Thompson. JAVMA 198(8) 4/15/91 pp1346-1347.

25. *Field of dreams: industrial veterinary medicine in the heart of Iowa.* Stephen Jaffe. JAVMA 199(6) 9/15/91 pp708-710.

26. *An idea whose time has come: Veterinarians in humane society administration.* Gary Patronek. JAVMA 202(6) 3/15/93 pp 862-864.

27. *Practice or perish? My path from practice to marketing to editing.* Tim Phillips. JAVMA 202(8) 4/15/93 pp 1222-1224.

INDEX

BOOK ORDERS

CAREER CHOICES FOR VETERINARIANS:
Beyond Private Practice

Smith Veterinary Services
Telephone orders: (509) 763-2052
Fax orders: (509) 763-2112
E-mail or online orders: smithvet@nwinternet.com
or 76206.3216@compuserve.com
http://www.now2000.com/smithvet
Mail Orders:
PO Box 254
Leavenworth WA 98826

Books are also available from
Veterinary Practice Publishing Company
213-385-2222 or 805-965-1028

ABOUT THE AUTHOR

Dr. Carin Smith is a veterinarian whose career paths include consultant, book author, and technical writer. She has written extensively on matters of concern and interest to veterinarians and the veterinary industry, as well as to owners of companion animals. Dr. Smith's books include three career guides for veterinarians and three pet care guides. She lives and works on a small farm in the mountains of Washington state.

Smith Veterinary Services
PO Box 254
Leavenworth WA 98826

Notes

Notes

Notes

Notes